Comprehensive Performance Nutrition

Quick Reference Q&A Guide

JUSTIN HARRIS

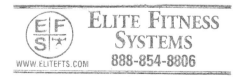

ELITE FITNESS SYSTEMS

WWW.ELITEFTS.COM   888-854-8806

"Success is not the key to happiness. Happiness is the key to success. If you love what you are doing, you will be successful."

Albert Schweitzer

Preface

My objective of this book is to present a comprehensive overview of performance-guided nutrition and training in an easy-to-follow question and answer format. I have spent much of my life learning and developing my interest in nutrition. I have often wished for an easy-to-follow guide that would allow me to continue my knowledge growth in brief time periods. I believe this book will provide much benefit to readers interested in developing their own knowledge base on training and nutrition. In this book, you will find definable answers to many real-world questions your peers have posed to me over the years.

Thank you to all those involved for your support.

CONTENTS

Performance Nutrition

The nutritional component of performance enhancement has long been a fascination of mine. Through many years of knowledge accumulation, I've come to one focused conclusion. There is a glaring shortage of nutritional information geared towards the performance-minded individual.

"Comprehensive Performance Nutrition" is a thorough compilation of true-life questions and answers to many issues regarding performance nutrition. This book is set up in an easy-to-read-and-comprehend question and answer format. This allows the reader to attain a full understanding of a particular issue in one brief session of reading. Each answer is straightforward and to-the-point, encompassing the question in a manner which allows the reader to have a firm grasp on the subject with a minimal investment of time.

"Comprehensive Nutrition" will allow you to further your understanding of nutrition and training as it pertains to the athlete's intent on improving his or her own performance.

Consider this your quick reference manual to many common questions regarding performance-geared nutrition and training.

FAT LOSS

Justin,

How exactly does fat loss occur in the body? Are there hormones or enzymes that do this? Is this how 'fat burners' work?

Fat loss is the physiologic process of Lipolysis. Lipolysis is the breakdown of the fat stored in fat cells. This causes the release of fatty acids into the bloodstream to circulate through the body. Ketones are also produced in this process.

Lipolysis is induced by:
Epinephrine: "adrenalin," both a hormone and a neurotransmitter.
Norepinephrine: Same as epinephrine, minus a methyl group.
Glucagon: Opposite of insulin. A hormone that causes glycogen to be released.
Adrenocorticotropin Hormone (ACTH): Released from the pituitary gland in response to stimuli.

All of these increase cAMP production.
      cAMP activates Protein Kinase A.
         Protein Kinase A activates Lipases.
Lipase: Main enzyme responsible for breaking down fats in humans.
cAMP is a second messenger, involved in signal transduction. It is necessary for hormones like glucagon and adrenalin (epinephrine and norepinephrine) to permeate cells.
When these fatty acids are released into the bloodstream, they can then be used for energy production by the body.

Justin,

I've been dieting since May 15th. I started at 205lbs and 20% body fat. I am currently 180lbs and 15% body fat. I've only used your methods for the past couple of weeks, but have concerns that my metabolism is shot from previous non-carb-cycling dieting. My goal is 200lbs at 10% body fat. I currently rotate 3 low days, 1 high, and 2 medium. My plan is to follow this until November 1st, gain for 8 weeks, and then diet again. Do you think I should continue on that long or take a break now?

Thanks.

Take a day and pig out. Eat as much as you can of whatever you want.

If you're sweating like crazy that night when you go to sleep, your metabolism will have had a kick start.

Get back on the carb rotation the next day.
If your body temperature ever feels like it is dropping, you need to kick start your metabolism again.

Justin,

In your recent article, "The Fat that Burns Fat," you were talking about GLA (linoleic acid) as a supplement. I currently use CLA (conjugated linoleic acid) as a supplement and on face value it looks like it's derived from the same sort of thing. Are GLA/CLA essentially the same thing?

The reason I ask is that one is a reasonably expensive supplement and the other is a lot cheaper product from a health store.

CLA is a different product.

CLA is actually a trans fat.
Much of the recent evidence on CLA shows little benefit to healthy, exercising people in regards to body fat loss.

GLA, or gamma-linolenic acid, is a derivative of Omega 6 fatty acids, which are essential to human life.
Linoleic acid, as you have written in your question, is different than GLA, although still an Omega 6 fatty acid.

Arachidonic acid, another derivative of Omega 6 fatty acids, is one of the most potent growth regulators of the body.

Omega 6 fatty acids are inflammatory and growth promoting.

I'm not a huge fan of CLA...although I feel the jury is still out on its benefits.

Justin,

Right now I'm "cutting." What's the best way to cook chicken? How do you give it flavor?

Grilling probably tastes the best...

Try this though:
Cut up all your chicken into a big pan and fill it up a bit with soy sauce and water until the chicken is covered.

Add salt, pepper, garlic salt, and maybe even some Asian or spicy sauce.

Cook on med-high heat on the stove top....just let it sit until the water cooks off. The chicken ends up being very moist and tender with a lot of flavor.

This method is very easy as well. There is no real need to stir the meat or look after it.
Once most of the water has boiled off, the meat should be ready to eat.

Dave Palumbo gave me the idea, and I've added a few things.

Justin,

Hey Justin, I'm a big fan. I'm a strongman competitor - right now I'm trying to get into better condition - I'm 30, 6' 278lbs. My body fat is under 20%, and I'd like to get leaner.

What's your take on milk? I gain mass quite easily (I've been 340lbs but was fat).

I make my shakes with 2 cups of skim milk - is this a mistake? Should I just make them with water and add a little EFA? Estrogen can creep up on me quite easily - water retention and body fat gain happen almost overnight with me.

Is milk a poor food choice?

I'd skip the milk.
Milk PROTEIN is an EXCELLENT nutrient source.

Milk CARBOHYDRATES aren't as great, in my opinion.

It is also important to note that liquid nutrients affect your appetite differently than solid food nutrients.
Evidence suggests that liquid calories cause different responses to ghrelin, one of the hunger hormones.

Our hunger is suppressed and increased in response to leptin, ghrelin, stomach 'stretching,' and also calorie intake.

Liquid calories are an easy way to increase nutrient intake when adding size.
I prefer to use waxy maize and specific amino acids in this purpose.

But if you gain body fat easily, I would suggest minimizing the amount of liquid calories you add to your meals. In other words, drop the milk.

If I have a protein shake in a carbohydrate meal, I'll typically have the protein alongside a carb source like oatmeal.

If I have a protein drink in a non-carb meal, I'll typically add natural peanut butter or another healthy form of fat for the fatty acids.

If anyone wants a good, quick breakfast that fosters an anabolic environment and tastes pretty good, try this:
1 scoop egg protein (or 1 cup egg whites)
1 scoop whey or casein protein
1/4-1/3 cup cashews (salted)
1 cup oats
Splenda to taste

Blend that with a lot of ice until it becomes a thick milkshake.

The cashews will make it taste creamy, like a milkshake.
You end up with a great amino acid mixture, great carb source (with SOLUBLE fiber), and healthy fats.

On a high day, drop the cashews down to 1/8th cup; add 2 cups oats, and some fruit or jelly.

Justin,

What is the lowest carb amount you would recommend on a low carb day? I'm about 170lbs at around 7-8% body fat. I want to try to get to about 4%. Would a 30g low day, 100g med day and 300g high day work?

30g low would be fine as long as you're careful to use healthy fats appropriately.

The 100g estimate is probably close, but you may be able to take it a bit higher.

I think you can get away with 400-500g on the high days if you're pushing the low and medium days hard enough.

Those amounts are going to be dependant on (and vary inversely to) your protein intake, so these are just estimates.

Justin,

Do you recommend that someone eats 3 meals and 3 snacks or 3 large meals? Would eating more meals increase metabolism?

It is probably most important to do what fits your schedule best and what allows you to be most consistent.

In the diets I give to clients, I typically have them eat 6-8 meals a day, depending on their body size and what the purpose of the plan is.

Each meal is roughly the same size, with meal 1 and post-workout possibly being higher in calories.

Justin,

I was reading a previous question you answered and I just wanted to make sure I understood the response correctly.

The more carbs you take in the less protein you need in a day?

And to prevent increased fat storage from all the carbs, I can raise my healthy fat intake?

Is that about how that would work with the carb cycling schedule?

Thanks.

Carbs increase insulin. On a receptor-to-receptor level, protein breakdown is impossible in the presence of insulin.

So when you eat more carbs, you don't need as much protein. And in fact, too much protein will just be stored as fat.

People think that when they eat 500g of protein, most of it is going to feed the muscles. If you converted 500g of protein to new muscle tissue each day, you'd be unfunctionably massive within the year.
It just doesn't work that way.

So it's not how much protein you eat, but how much you can synthesize into new muscle tissue.

When your carb intake is high, your protein intake can be much lower...and even though it is lower, you can get MORE synthesis of new muscle, as you will be converting MUCH less protein to glucose...leaving more available for synthesis of muscle.

DO NOT increase healthy fat intake on high carb days though. Insulin is a storage hormone...eat a ton of carbs, and take in fat with it, and you will just store the fat as fat.

On the lower carb days, you can increase healthy fat intake. Omega 3 fatty acids increase insulin sensitivity making your cells (muscle cells) more sensitive to insulin, requiring less insulin to perform the necessary nutrient shuffling.

By increasing healthy fat intake on the low carb days, you can deplete muscle glycogen stores a bit, while also increasing insulin sensitivity of the cells.

Then when you take in the carbs on high carb days, you have the potential for super-compensation of muscle glycogen and more efficient uptake and utilization of protein and carbs because of the increase in insulin sensitivity.

When carb intake goes up....protein and fat intake should go down. When protein and fat go up...carbs go down.

Justin,

I asked about cutting weight earlier. I have not done anything with my sodium intake. I do not add a lot to my food so how would I drop my sodium and how far out would you start dropping?

Thanks.

It may be too late, but I would begin adding more sodium to my food a few weeks before the show.
When sodium is added to your food, your body changes its production of Aldosterone.

High blood sodium concentration will tell your body to lower production of Aldosterone.
Aldosterone increases sodium reabsorption in the distal tubule of the kidney. So when its production is lowered, sodium is excreted more rapidly.

What ends up happening is that even though you're eating more salt, you stop holding extra water.
Then, about 72 hours before the weigh-ins, you lower sodium intake and your body continues to flush higher amounts of sodium from the body, despite the fact that you aren't eating as much.

Then, and this is important for powerlifting meets, your body senses the lowered sodium concentration and increases Aldosterone production.
This doesn't affect you yet however, because you're still eating low sodium.

Another thing that happens is, when you get dehydrated, and your blood vessels shrink from lack of fluid, stretch receptors in the blood vessels sense the lack of fluid and also tell your body to pump out Aldosterone.
So when you finally make weight, your body is primed to store

sodium, and that sodium will force your body to retain fluids.

So after making weight, you re-introduce sodium, water, and carbohydrates, and you've set yourself up as a glycogen-storing, water-hoarding machine.

If done properly, this will allow you to be re-hydrated, fully glycogen loaded, and stuffed with intracellular and extracellular water stores to fuel you during the meet.

DISCLAIMER:
Clearly, this isn't the healthiest approach for your body...it would be safer to be under weight to begin with and not have to deal with all this stuff.

But in an age when people resort to diuretics and other harmful tricks to make weight, this is a way for you to work with your body's OWN mechanisms to both make weight and re-stock for the meet.

Justin,

If someone has done too much cardio too early in the diet (Palumbo's keto diet in my case) and would want to reverse the tendency, what strategy would be best to keep losing fat while somehow resetting the metabolism?

Related to the previous question, are there any rules concerning metabolism, e.g. 1 week without cardio to reset cardio tolerance, etc? In brief, how do you keep maximum cardio efficiency?

In "The Keto Diet" by Lyle McDonald, he states that if your calorie deficit (food deficit and exercise expenditure combined) is too low, metabolism will slow down: "This threshold occurs at approximately 1000 calories per day below maintenance and represents the maximum allowed deficit." What are your thoughts on this?

In reverse:

The body aims to maintain homeostasis. It doesn't like burning fat because low fat stores means you won't survive a famine.

So, go too low in calories for too long, and your metabolism will slow down to prevent total loss of body fat.

As for the 1,000 calories...I don't like absolutes when it comes to the body. The human body just has too many variables, but I would bet at that amount you will see metabolic lag for sure.

Don't worry about cardio tolerance. Do the cardio and follow the diet. If you become more tolerant to cardio, you can be happy knowing your cardiovascular system is healthier.
If you're tracking your heart rate response to exercise, just increase cardio intensity as needed to keep your heart rate in your target range.

How much is too much cardio?
If you were too excited and started doing 2 hours of cardio a day at the start of the diet....just remember that there is no real way to rush progress. Keep pushing forward and always try to improve. Don't search for a magic bullet.

It will be pretty tough to back down cardio drastically without changing the diet, and still burn fat. It will be even more difficult to make those changes and continue burning fat at the same rate. You can try tapering cardio slowly and slowly reducing caloric intake to match the negative calorie loss from the cardio.

If you're doing a contest, you may not have time to play with all those things, and you might have to bite the bullet and over-cardio it right through the show.

Justin,

In carb cycling diets, do you generally aim to keep total calories relatively constant across the high, medium, and low days, adjusting only fat and protein in accordance with the changes in carb levels for those days? Or do low and medium carb days also mean lower total calories than the high days?

Thanks.

The calorie count typically varies in some proportion to the carb amount.

While fat and protein will be a bit lower on high carb days, the calorie total will still be higher.

For dieting, low and medium days are hypo-caloric days (below your metabolic rate) and high days are hyper-caloric days (above your basal metabolic rate).

For adding size, the only day that is potentially hypo-caloric is low day, and even then it is often higher than your BMR.

Justin,

Is low intensity cardio only productive when you are low on carbs? Because when I wasn't dieting, I tried powerwalking in the morning on an empty stomach 3-4 times a week, 45 minutes each time, and noticed nothing in the way of fat loss? I just wore myself out for the weights!

Thanks for your time.

Richard

Richard,
Low intensity cardio actually burns a higher percentage of calories from fat compared to high intensity cardio.
So it is an effective fat burner.

The problem is that the total calories burned with low intensity cardio are very minimal. So despite the fact that a high *percentage* of fat is burned compared to total calories burned, the *total* calories are still pretty low.

I personally prefer moderate to high intensity cardio for longer durations. I like to work hard when I do cardio, but not drain myself.

A funny tidbit...the time of day you're most efficient at fat burning is actually during sleep.
So, why can't you just sleep away the fat?

Because despite the fact that you burn a very high *percentage* of calories from fat during sleep, the *total* calorie amount burned is very low.

Justin,

If I go for a super high carb day every once in a while, how high should I go and how much protein would you take out on that day? My protein, carb, fat breakdown right now is roughly...
Low - 250, 150, 150
Med - 225, 300, 100
High - 200, 450, 70

I weigh about 215 lbs. I'm thinking of going to 600g carbs on this day and dropping protein to about 175g, with fat intake less than 50g.

Thanks,
Scott

You can probably up the carbs to 600g, and if they're that high, you can definitely get by with 175g protein.

Remember that with 600g of carbs, your blood sugar and insulin levels will be elevated all day...this means that on a receptor-to-receptor basis, muscle loss is impossible...

So even though you're eating less protein, it could be argued that more protein is available for adding muscle on this day.

Of course, with the high carb intake, you're at more risk for fat storage and you have to be diligent with your meals, but that is why we have the lower carb days.

You may want to lower fat to about 100g on the low day as well. With fat that high, there will be less need to use stored glycogen as energy. You want to be mildly glycogen depleted leading into the high days to set up the potential for super-compensation of glycogen stores.

Justin,

I'm trying to lose a significant amount of weight over the next year, but don't want to sacrifice my strength. I've heard people say doing cardio can cause strength gains to stop. My questions are, if cardio is necessary, what type should I do? How often should I do it? Or will most of the weight loss come from diet adjustments? Secondly, is it possible to still put on muscle while losing fat? I apologize for the lengthiness of the question, and thanks for your advice.

I'm doing 2 hours of cardio a day right now.
I just hit 600x5 and 635x3 on squats, as well as 855x4 on rack deads.

Assuming an increase in cardiovascular fitness will make you weaker is a false assumption in my opinion.

If you don't lose the muscle, you shouldn't lose the strength.

I tell people to make adjustments to help keep intra and extra cellular fluid levels high in order to maintain better leverages across your joints.
I do this by maintaining a high sodium intake throughout the diet.

In fact, you can see in Dave Tate's recent log that even at 4% body fat he was able to handle the same weights as he was at 13% body fat when he kept sodium intake high.

If you believe you will lose strength, you will. If you understand that you haven't lost muscle, you should understand that you don't have to lose strength.

I prefer moderate intensity, and moderate to long duration cardio.
I use the stepmill and a steep incline treadmill.

Justin,

I am a 265lb football player who is using your carb cycling protocols to lower my weight to 255 by the end of July.

My questions are:
1) What do you think of the following approach? I have 5 low carb days/week, 1 medium carb day, and 1 high carb day. I will change a scheduled low-carb day to a medium carb or even a high carb day if my training feels compromised. I consider myself pretty in-tune with my body and know what to look for.
2) On the high carb day, I will have trouble getting to 800g if I use all fibrous carbs. I know Dave Tate has written about how he used sugared cereal as half of his carbs on one such day. If I am trying to shock my metabolism and plan on eating around every hour, how "dirty" can these carbs be? I'm not talking about pounding Gatorades all day, but flavored oatmeal packets? Cereal? My medium carb day consists of all fibrous, low-glycemic carbs. I vary my fat and protein intake according to carb intake in a manner very similar to what you recommend.

Thanks for any insight you can offer,
Tim

That is much different than I typically approach diets.

I typically rotate carbs in a high, med, low rotation.

In someone of your size, even if you're carrying a good deal of body fat, I would never have you go under 30g of carbs a day. I would probably not have you go under 100g per day.

The problem with 5 days of a carb intake that low is that you're not really doing a carb rotation diet. You're setting yourself up to go into ketosis, a state in which the body does not have enough blood sugar to fuel normal brain function, and thus uses ketones to fuel the brain function.

If you are doing a ketogenic diet (which what you have listed more closely resembles), I would recommend a cheat meal instead of a high carb day.

When you have the high carb day in your current setting, you kick yourself out of ketosis for up to 3 days. During this time you will feel very weak and sluggish. Then, just as you get back into ketosis, you're throwing carbs back in, which knocks you back out of ketosis.

If you have a cheat meal, you are kicked out of ketosis for hours instead of days.

If you follow my dieting approach, carbs remain the main fuel for weight training and the brain, so a high carb day refuels glycogen stores and amps up the metabolism. We're not in ketosis, so it isn't a concern.

Justin,

Do your nutritionists lay out exactly what foods and supplements to eat, when to eat them, and how much to eat?

Also, how do they monitor progress and make adjustments? I'm looking at the progressive plan and looking to go from about 215lbs and 20% body fat to about 200lbs and 15% body fat and then hopefully 200lbs and 10% body fat. At that point, I'd be looking to focus more on strength training like I've done in the past.

I just feel like I've let myself get too far out of shape right now and I also have some mobility issues to work through. Does this sound like something one of your guys could help with?

Scott

Our nutritionists detail everything in regards to diet, fat loss supplements (or whatever your particular plan entails), and cardio work.
They offer any training advice that the client wishes as well.

We monitor and change the plan based on how you respond through your correspondence with the nutritionist, as well as from your weekly photo check ups.

Your plan is very reasonable and I think you'll find our nutritionists would be able to get you a great deal further than you ask here.

Justin,

First I wanted to say awesome video and the nutrition DVD is great. My question is: Would you count the carbs in something such as V-8 or a greens type drink?

Thanks for the info,

Adam

I really try to never drink calories. So yes, I would count the carbs in V-8 for sure.
As for the greens drink, if there are 5 calories or less per serving, I wouldn't count them. If there are more than 5 calories per serving, count the calories.

Justin,

Do the nutritionists on your website do diet plans the way you would?

Yes, they all set up diets exactly the same as me.
They are all clients of mine, have been for years, and know how I do things.

We all keep in touch via email so they know and understand the new techniques I begin to use.
There is always room to improve the dieting process, so we all share information, studies we find, and techniques we use.

I trust them for my own diet changes and ask their critiques and input for myself when dieting.

Justin,

I need help with my nutrition. I'm a 37-year-old male, 6'2" and 340lbs. I want to get down to about 280lbs. I'm healthy so far and I get a physical every year. My sugar, blood pressure, thyroid, and cholesterol are all fine. I do have sleep apnea and sleep with a CPAP machine. I know I need to lose weight and I'm working on it. I now have a position sitting behind a desk (makes it harder to lose).

I try to eat right—nothing fried, just baked. I try to eat 6 times a day and I consume protein shakes. Most meals are baked chicken or tuna fish, brown rice (slow burning carb) and corn or green beans. I do use creatine, multivitamin, and ZMa. I also use a fat burner (Lipo-6) and before I work out I take EAS Muscle Armor and No-Xplode. My problem is that I stay tired most of the time. I get 8 hours of sleep (in bed by 9:30 p.m. and up at 5:30 a.m.). Since I'm on 1st shift (7 a.m. to 3 p.m.) I drink about 2 cups of coffee during the day. When I get ready to work out at 3:30 p.m. sometimes I'm out of gas even though I took the No-Xplode and Lipo-6! I tried going without the coffee but I get so sleepy. I'm trying to stay around 2500 calories a day. Do I need more calories per day? If so, please tell me how many. Your knowledge would be greatly appreciated. I know you're busy, but HELP!!!

Jody

Jody,
That is probably a good calorie amount on your 'medium' carb days.

Make sure you're rotating your carbs in a high, medium, and low fashion.

Take your calories higher on heavy training days, moderate on other training days, and bring them very low on off days.

You're eating the right foods; you just need to be consistent. People don't get to 300lbs in a month, so don't expect to lose the weight in a month.

Consistency is key.
Most Americans eat pretty close to their maintenance calorie level each day.

Most Americans don't pig out each day. But, Americans tend to gain a pound of fat during the holidays (yes....only a pound of fat...which they NEVER lose, and in 25 years, becomes 25 pounds of fat).

Then, during the summer months, they will have a few barbecues a month where they put down a ton of calories from junk. This results in another few pounds gained each year.

Then, during the winter, they get less exercise and are more tempted to stay in the house at night eating junk. This results in another few pounds gained each year.

These MINOR things add up to an easy 10 pounds a year, which over 10 years can be 100 pounds of added weight, done without ever thinking you were over-eating!

Consistency is key.

Justin,

I've noticed you normally have 2 low carb days in a row when setting up carb cycling diets. Is this necessary? The reason I ask is because of my training split. For instance, my training split goes like this:
Monday - ME Bench
Tuesday - Off
Wednesday - ME SQ/DL
Thursday - DE Bench
Friday - Off
Saturday - DE SQ
Sunday - Off

I was thinking of trying out the carb cycling and with that split I was thinking of this:
Monday - Moderate
Tuesday - Low
Wednesday - High
Thursday - Moderate
Friday - Low
Saturday - Moderate
Sunday - Low

Currently I'm a powerlifter, 320lbs, higher body fat than I'd like to admit, and am looking to drop fat and get stronger. Thanks in advance and thank you for all the nutritional advice you've been handing out. It really makes a difference!

You set it up how I would set it up with your rotation.

I actually don't like to have two low days in a row if possible.

The ideal rotation in my opinion is to have it set up in a roughly high, med, low rotation.

But, I do like to have high days on heavy training days and low days on off days, so it will depend on your personal training schedule.

How you have it set up is perfect. You should be able to hold, or even gain, strength and lose body fat very steadily.

Justin,

Several weeks ago I submitted my nutrition plan for you to review. I've reached a plateau and so here are my ideas for staggering my carbs:

High carb days
MEAL 1
1 serving plain oats
3 servings Egg Beaters
1 serving skim milk
1 piece of fruit or 1 slice whole grain bread
multivitamin
MEAL 2 (usually pre-workout)
2 slices whole grain bread
6 oz. turkey breast
small can of V-8
MEAL 3 (post-workout)
Myoplex original shake
1 slice whole grain bread
1 Tbsp jelly
MEAL 4
1 serving non-fat cottage cheese
2 servings cherries or pineapple in cottage cheese
MEAL 5
1 large chicken breast
1 sweet potato or 2 servings whole wheat pasta
3-4 servings vegetables
MEAL 6 (only if I am hungry later in the evening)
handful of boiled peanuts

Low carb days
MEAL 1
4 servings Egg Beaters
2 Tbsp natural peanut butter
MEAL 2
2 servings non-fat cottage cheese
MEAL 3 (post cardio)

Myoplex Lite shake
MEAL 4
1 can of tuna with mustard
small can of V-8
6 oz. turkey breast
MEAL 5
2 veggie burgers w/ ketchup and mustard
MEAL 6
1 large chicken breast
3-4 servings of vegetables
MEAL 7
2 servings non-fat cottage cheese

With my training, everything looks like this:
Monday - HIGH CARB, bench, triceps accessory, weighted
pull-ups, abs, 25 minutes HIIT
Tuesday - LOW CARB, 20-30 minutes swimming
Wednesday - HIGH CARB, incline bench, deadlift,
hamstrings, bicep accessory, 25 minutes HIIT
Thursday - LOW CARB
Friday - HIGH CARB, squats, lower back, calves, barbell rows
or lat pull-downs, 25 minutes HIIT

I'm 6'4" and I'm now down to 244lbs. I'm not sure about my
body fat percentage because I haven't been able to get anyone
to check it for me. My strength is still going up, although very
slowly, and so I feel like I'll still be able to compete in
Strongman/PL while dieting.

Looks pretty good, actually.
I don't like the veggie burgers, and I'm not a huge fan of milk.
When trying to lose body fat, I prefer less fruit and refined
carbohydrates.
But, your amounts and the set up and rotation look good. I would
guess that if you begin stagnating, you will need to move your carb
sources around a bit to a less sugary type, but otherwise you should
be able to continue to add strength while you lean out.

Justin,

I have a mindset and a goal right now to lose some body fat and get a bit leaner. I'm 5'7" and weigh 215lbs at around 20% body fat. I would like to get down to around 185-195lbs, yet be low in body fat. I can honestly say that my diet right now sucks! I tend to eat stuff like fast food, pizza, soda, beer, and other junk. What kind of diet foods would you suggest that I eat instead? Also what kind of conditioning can I do that will help me drop my body fat levels? I train Westside style.

Thanks.

Change the eating.
If you can't pick it, grow it, or kill it...don't eat it.
You don't go hunting for pizza. You don't pick beer from trees (that happens in heaven), and you don't grow soda in the soda fields.

Each meal should contain a steady amount of protein from lean sources, a complex carb source, and healthy fats.

Rotate your carbs and your calories each day and continue to train heavy.

Any conditioning training will help burn fat. Anything that burns calories had the potential to burn fat. Just get moving.

Justin,

Hi, I've been reading up on your carb cycling diet. I'm a powerlifter but I'm trying to stay closer to my competition weight. I've never seen the point of trying to drop water weight before a meet and still carrying around an extra 10 to 15 pounds of fat. Right now I'm about 185lbs and around 12% body fat. I'd like to bring up my lean mass while dropping down to about 8% BF. I train in the evening on Tuesdays and Wednesdays. The diet is easy on those days, but on Saturday and Sunday I have to train earlier. How would I cycle my calories on those days since I'm training around noon?

Easy.
Make the off days low carb days.
Make your two heaviest days high carb days, and make the other two days medium days.

You don't need the carbs on your off days. You're not fueling any training.
Keep the protein high and the healthy fats moderate so you're able to grow and recover from the other training days.

On the days you train earlier, you're probably even better off. By training in the a.m., you get more meals after your workout to aid in recovery.

Justin,

First of all, thanks for all of your nutritional advice. It seems fairly easy to understand and even easier to follow.

Now, onto the question. This is geared towards a diet designed to drop body fat percentage. I noticed that with most diets you have outlined in the Q&A that the fat levels seem very low. I know with the super high carb days to keep them next to zero due to a couple factors, but on your low and medium carb days I'm guessing the fats are below 40g each day, with some number crunching I'm thinking it's around 20-30g a day in healthy fats.

Am I right here? Or am I mixing something up?

If so, without revealing all of your secrets, what's the reasoning behind it? For some reason, I've always read and have been told that fats should be higher on lower carb days than high carb days. I've also read that this fat is important for our joints.

Thanks in advance.

The fat levels are much higher than that in my diets.

Today is a low day for me and I will probably have around 100g of fats throughout the day. Some of that will be in addition to what is found in my protein sources and some of that will be extra fat added to the meals.

Justin,

I read earlier where you said to have a low, medium, and high carb day. I was wondering what the purpose of the medium carb day is, and how do you fit it into your rotation?

Medium carb days are for dieting. I typically only have high carb and 'normal' carb days in the offseason.

The medium carb day is a day where fat burning is still highly likely, but calories are high enough to efficiently fuel weight training.

They also help maintain a higher resting metabolic rate, at least in my experience.

Justin,

What is the significance of medium carb days? Can one just do low carb days and high carb days?

Yeah, you can do just low and high carb days.
The medium days are just another way to keep your metabolism elevated, and keep you from getting too flat.

I've done things both ways. I find people are able to keep size better, and get in shape easier, with the medium days. Less high days are needed and fat burning is still very high on the medium days.

Justin,

This may be sweating the details, but do you count carbs from fruit and vegetables towards the daily carb counts?

Thanks in advance.

Fruit is made up primarily of simple sugars. Many fruits are quite high in calories and carbohydrates. If you were to avoid counting the carbs in one large banana, you would miss 30g of carbs and over 100 calories. That is certainly enough to create a noticeable difference in your physique over time.

I don't count most vegetables.
Green leafy vegetables are low enough in carbs and high enough in fiber for me to typically consider them a 'free' food.

This free food moniker is only for leafy green vegetables though. Higher carb vegetables like green beans or corn would count towards your daily total.

But, lettuce typically has about 3g of carbs per fairly large serving, of which 2g is fiber. So it is very likely that you will BURN more than the 1g of 'true' carbs in the lettuce just from eating and digesting it.

I have, however, run into a few people who go WAY overboard with the "free" vegetables outlet.

I had one girl who was eating 40 asparagus stalks a meal.
That is definitely overboard. Dieting is a time of LESS food intake. It is not a time to be a gluttonous pig. But for some people, the word "free food" turns them into total gluttons.

Justin,

What do you think of the Anabolic Diet? It's basically low carb from Monday to Friday and then high carb on the weekends. Would this be a decent carb cycling approach?

It depends on a few factors.

If the goal of the anabolic diet is to get into ketosis, you're going to be dealing with energy source struggles. It becomes kind of a 'dueling banjos' between the brain relying on glucose and relying on ketones.

It can take 3 days to get into the state of ketosis where the brain begins using ketones for fuel. In this approach, assuming the carbs are low enough, fat is high enough, and protein isn't too high, you will be in ketosis around Wednesday after the high carb weekends.

This will create high levels of insulin sensitivity, which will cause increased levels of glycogen storage over the higher carb weekends.

The problem then is, after 2 days of carbs, you are out of ketosis, and the body is using glucose as its brain fuel. So on Monday, Tuesday, and probably some of Wednesday, your brain is saying "huh?" and looking for glucose, and it isn't getting much. This will leave you feeling less than stellar. Then Wednesday, you're back into ketosis, only to do it all over again.

My personal feelings on very low carb diets is they can be effective, and you can feel quite good. Essential fatty acids produce some nice "feel good" actions in the body, such as less inflammation, cushioned joints, high essential fatty acid reserves in the muscle, steady blood sugar levels, etc.

But, the back and forth between glucose and ketones for the brain may leave you feeling odd a few days each week.

If I were to use a low carb diet, I would either keep carbs very low, just incidentals from the nuts I would eat, using moderate healthy fat levels, and moderate to high protein levels, with a huge cheat meal once a week. This "cheat meal" will take you out of ketosis, but most likely only for a period of a few hours.

Or, I would use a moderate to high protein intake, moderate fat intake, and low to moderate carb intake, with the bulk of carbs coming around my workouts.

I would still probably utilize a cheat meal once a week.

Justin,

What's your take on fruit as a carbohydrate source?

Shelby

Shelby,
I'm not a huge fan of fruit as a carbohydrate source. I don't really think it is as bad as many people want to make it out to be, however.

Fructose, a main sugar in fruit, isn't the 'greatest' carb source for what we want to accomplish in bodybuilding.

But, fructose isn't the ONLY carb source in fruit. Some fruits actually have higher amounts of dextrose than fructose, if I remember correctly. And when you add in any fiber, along with the vitamins and minerals, fruit has many benefits.

One often overstated misconception about fructose is that it can 'only' be stored as liver glycogen.
This isn't true.
Fructose can and will be stored as muscle glycogen.
Its initial storage will usually be more predicated to liver storage, as the liver is what controls blood sugar levels, but fructose will be stored in muscle tissue as well.

In fact, in a glycogen-depleted state, one could argue the possibility that fructose is good for restoring glycogen, as it will only be more predisposed for muscle glycogen storage in a muscle glycogen-depleted state, and at the point when muscle glycogen levels are beginning to reach effective levels of fullness, the fructose has another viable option of storage in the liver....don't know if you'll find any studies on that though.

But, you can find studies showing some BENEFITS of muscle glycogen storage with fructose.

One particular study examining the effects of fructose intake (20% of the diet...a high amount of pure fructose as a total percentage of the diet) found this result: "These results indicate that both long-term intake of the fructose diet and exercise training synergistically increased glycogen in both tissues."

So, long term intake of a high fructose diet showed higher glycogen levels in the liver AND muscle.

Justin,

When dieting, do you still use the pre- and during-workout shakes...maybe without the carbs? Also, what are your feelings on mixing whey and casein post-workout as some studies/magazines now suggest?

Thanks!

When dieting, I tend to stick to 6 meals per day, with almost all of them being whole food meals.
My goals switch when I am dieting. I am no longer specifically looking to be anabolic around my workouts.
My main goal is to be anti-catabolic.

I stick to more whole food protein sources and slow digesting carb sources, even post-workout.

I think whey and casein are a fine combo post-workout, especially if you are not going to eat another meal within 90 minutes of a whey-only shake.

Studies regarding training and human physiology are going to have a high risk for flaws, as little is often considered of the patient's diet prep outside of the small window of time they record.

Justin,

I have some questions in regards to a consistently low carb diet. I am an athlete who about 2 years ago discovered the principles to the conjugate method and then shortly thereafter utilized them. Within the first year without much rotation of exercises I was able to add 50 pounds to my bench and 65 pounds to my squat, but most importantly was running the 40 in consistent 4.4's. The amazing part about it is I really don't have that young of a conditioning age. Anyway, for the last 3 months or so I have been in quite a bit of a rut, and everything seemed to drop off a bit. I focused for a minute on conditioning thinking it may have been a hindering factor. The only thing that has shown progress is my agilities times due to the body fat I have dropped. This brings me to my diet. I am 5'11 and 206lbs currently. My body fat is around 6% (5.8). I basically started eating clean and cut out rice, pasta, and bread. I get most of my carbs from fruits and vegetables, along with dried fruit and salads. I have tried doing less, which did work for awhile, but my question to you is will this hinder my progress? Please note I also have had some trouble sleeping lately. I am wondering if these items may be affecting the development of the nervous system. I look like I have always wanted to, but is this at the expense of performance? Any help you could lend is greatly appreciated. Also, if you could, would you advise on high and low days for someone carb-sensitive with my dimensions.

Thank you!

I'm not a huge fan of fruit carb sources. If you're eating a very regimented diet with the proper amount of healthy fats each meal, you can create a steady blood glucose level with the simple carbs. But if anything is off, you're going to have swings in blood sugar levels that will throw off your energy and performance ability.

For what you have listed here, and this will have to be a

generalization as I don't have a ton of history on you, I would plan on something like this for the diet:

Make sure you're getting protein and vegetables in every meal. The protein is necessary, as there is a constant turnover of nitrogen in the body.
The vegetables will give you healthy nutrients and fiber to slow digestion of the carbohydrates you ingest.

I would start with just a high and low carb day. You can add in a medium day at a later time.

On the low day, keep carbs pretty low. To keep body fat that low (which is pretty low), you will probably want to stay around 100g of carbs per day. This isn't including the carbs in the vegetables or the carbs in any fat sources you may take in.

So that would be something along the order of 35g in 3 meals, or 25g in 4 meals.

In any meal where you don't have carbs, add some healthy fats. These should come from mostly nuts, natural peanut butter, borage oil, evening primrose oil, or fish oil.

Limit yourself to about 5g of additional fat in those meals.

Your high days should be focused on your training, having around 2 of them per week. These should be either the day of, or the day before, an intense training day.

Lower protein a bit in each meal and limit fats as much as possible. Load up on good, complex carbs from sources that contain little fat.
I don't like a ton of sugar on this day either.

You can probably plan on around 400-500g of carbs on this day, depending on how intense your training will be. Spread those carbs out over the course of the day.

Justin,

I am currently doing high-intensity cardio for about 20-30 minutes 4 times a week for fat loss. I am a student and I work so I don't have time to make two trips to the gym a day. Because of this I do my cardio right after my workout. Would you suggest I drink my post-workout shake after my workout before I hit the cardio or wait until I have finished the cardio? Thanks and good luck with your contest prep.

Sean

I wait until I've finished my cardio.

I also do my cardio post-workout. If you take in your post-workout shake before doing the cardio, you're setting up a situation where you have the nutrients available to fuel your cardio session, and you have not utilized stored fat as much as you could.

If your post-workout shake has carbs, and specifically 'fast' carbs (simple sugars), you will be getting a spike in insulin levels from that shake. High insulin levels raise an enzyme in your body that tells the mitochondria NOT to burn fat for energy.

To top it off, you will have used much of the nutrients in that shake to fuel your cardio session and will be in need of new nutrients to create an anabolic environment from your weight training.

Don't worry about losing muscle. People worry way too much about this in my opinion. The human body doesn't disintegrate from a short walk.

Save the shake for after the cardio. It will help you recover from both your training and your cardio.

Justin,

I want to start dieting using your carb cycling idea. I know you can't go into too much detail since this is your job, but what do you think about the following:
High Carb Days: 500g carbs, 250g protein
Med Carb Days: 250g carbs, 300g protein
Low Carb Days: 65g carbs, 400g protein

Currently I am 6'3" 275lbs, probably around 20% body fat. Do these numbers look about right and how much fat should I add on each of these days? How many total calories should I shoot for each of these days? Thanks!

That looks pretty good; perhaps a bit low in protein on the med day for my liking. You could increase carbs or protein on that day, but it isn't far off at all, so don't change much.

On the low day, you could plan on eating about 5g or so of healthy fat per meal.

I prefer evening primrose oil, borage oil, cashews, macadamia nut oil, natural peanut butter, and almonds.

I really prefer the first two options, but the other ones taste better, and 5g per meal isn't a whole lot of food to add.

Justin,

What kind of diet plan would you have someone follow if their goal was to lose body fat, but maintain/gain muscle mass? I know you have to eat a lot to gain muscle, but my problem is that I'm gaining more fat than muscle. My goal right now is to lose some body fat and get leaner. My workout routine is working each muscle group once a week. Hope you can help me!

Thanks.

You can only gain muscle so fast.

Theoretically, you have to eat more than you burn to synthesize new muscle tissue.
People tend to think of this as a day-to-day process, but protein turnover is a continuous process, so in reality, it is a minute-by-minute process.

This means you constantly have the chance to add muscle, lose muscle, gain fat, lose fat, etc., etc.

Attempting to pig out in order to gain new muscle is pointless and can be counter-productive in the long run.

Something that I like to have people do is follow 1-3 VERY high carb days each week.

On these days, carbohydrates will be VERY high, and insulin levels will be elevated throughout the day.
Insulin has many effects on the body. It is obviously a storage hormone, but is just as effective at storing fat as it is at storing carbohydrates.
So on this day, fat is kept to a minimum.

Insulin is HIGHLY anti-catabolic, so it will be essentially

physiologically impossible on a cell-to-cell basis to utilize protein for energy.

This means that a much higher percentage of protein you eat that day will be available for synthesis of new muscle tissue. So even though you're eating less protein....MORE protein will be available for synthesis of new muscle.

Now, the body has a very definite limit to the amount of glycogen it can store, and once you reach that point, further hyper-caloric and high carbohydrate dietary intake can lead to fat gain.

So, we lower carbohydrates and increase protein intake on the other days of the week.

These days will still provide high protein intake, which should be adequate to create new muscle mass at an efficient rate.

Carbohydrate levels are lower, but we have high levels of glycogen stored to fuel our training and workouts.

On these days, we may actually eat less calories than we burn, and since insulin levels will be lower, we create a potential environment where fat stores may need to be used for energy.

Insulin has some other interesting actions as well. It is a mild CNS depressant, which can help explain why you may feel sluggish after a very high carb meal or during a very high carb day.

Insulin decreases SHBG (steroid hormone binding globulin), which is what is responsible for binding to steroid hormones (IE: YOUR TESTOSTERONE PRODUCTION) and rendering it "bound" or inactive.

Insulin increases GFR, which means it is a mild diuretic. So you may feel like you're urinating more on high carb days.

Insulin increases sodium reabsorption, which means you may look bloated from sodium retention and subsequent water retention the day after a high carb day.

Justin,

I am 27, 265lbs and about 21% body fat. I am training for strongman and would like to drop my body fat down while getting stronger. I have been able to drop about 50lbs so far by using my own plan (with help! basically a low carb and high protein type thing). But, my strength has dropped off quite a bit with the weight loss.

I have done my research on this website and here is what I have put together so far:

Sun- low carb, .25g/#lbm, protein 2g/#lbm- yoga

Mon- moderate carb 1g/#lbm, protein 1.5g/#lbm- upper body

Tues- moderate- lower body

Wed- low carb- 1 hour cardio

Thurs- moderate carb- upper body

Fri- low carb- cardio

Sat- high carb- 2g/#lbm carbs, 1g/#lbm protein- strongman events

I usually take 1T of fish oil per day and try to limit the fat I get from other sources. So, add some veggies to the above plan, and this is the diet I am going to try. Do you think this is a good plan to try to get my strength up while losing fat, and fat only?

Yeah, that looks like a good plan.

You may find that you will need another high day during the week every few weeks.

You will need to let your "flatness" be your guide, and not your hunger though.

On that plan, what you're doing essentially is creating saturated glycogen stores on the high day, which will allow you to have available fuel on the low and medium days.

On the low days, carbs are very low, which should allow you to utilize a higher level of fat for energy.

On medium days, carbs are a bit higher to help fuel intense training.

And then, just as you are about to get too depleted and have your strength levels drop, you have the high day to re-saturate glycogen stores.

The difficulty in these situations is knowing when to change the diet around, adding high days, lowering carbs, switching med days to low days, etc.

But, the base set-up is good, and you should notice good changes!

Good luck.

Justin,

I've been doing DC for about a year now with great results. I'm currently using the 3-way split for recovery reasons.

I'm 5'10" and about 270lbs with around 20% body fat. I'm an insulin dependant diabetic, which complicates things for me.

I changed my diet to high protein (500-600 grams/day) and low carb with a few cheat meals a week. Since doing this, I've gained about 10 lbs of muscle. I've also lost enough fat to have stretch marks and loose skin. However, as of late, the fat loss has slowed down.
I'm curious how you deal with fat loss for diabetics.

Thanks.

Insulin blunts fatty acid transfer to the mitochondria; this is one way that insulin blunts energy utilization from fat stores. A biotin driven enzyme derivative of Acetyl CoA called Acetyl CoA Carboxylase II is primarily involved in this process.
This blunting of fatty acid transfer to the mitochondria is dose-dependant; as more insulin is produced, more receptors will be saturated, and greater number of mitochondria will be affected.

You can never totally eliminate insulin levels in the body. What we want to do is create low, steady levels of insulin.

If you eat a lower carb diet, you should be able to adjust your daily insulin amount.

But, many people lower carb intake, and then replace it by LOADING up extra protein. Extra protein will be converted to glucose, which then raises blood sugar levels all over again.

With insulin dependant diabetics (assuming they have the auto-immune disease of the pancreas, and not type II diabetics who have regressed to needing insulin in addition to oral diabetic meds), you can approach diet in a similar manner as if you aren't an insulin dependant diabetic.

Focus on good, healthy, essentially fatty acids in amounts that are inversely proportional to your carbohydrate intake.

Focus on good, complete protein sources.

And rotate your carb amounts.
I prefer to utilize a rotation of high carb days, medium carb days, and low carb days.

You need to be precise with your insulin and monitor your blood sugar very closely.

Please be careful not to skip insulin injections to lower insulin levels in the body. The body must have available glucose when exercising. If you skip an injection believing it will speed up fat loss, your body will struggle to find the sugar it needs, which can result in keto-acidosis.

Take it slowly, and learn how your body responds to the various amounts of carbs each day.

Justin,

How do I contact you to hire you for diet help?

Thanks.

Anyone that is interested in working with me, any of our nutritionists, or in purchasing our products, visit us at www.TroponinNutrition.com

OFFSEASON DIETING

Justin,

I am currently using a carb rotation to put on mass while minimizing fat gain, utilizing high and low carb days. If my workouts are at around 7-8pm, and I go to sleep around 11:30pm (so I get 2 meals after training, not including shake), should I keep carbs elevated for the first few meals of the following day? And how close to a workout can I raise carbs? 1 hour before? More? Less?

Thanks.

If you eat carbs after a hard workout, they're likely to be properly utilized no matter how close it is to bed.

The next day will be many hours after the workout, so don't worry about that.

Have high days on your heaviest training days, and lower carb days on the other days. Growth occurs at all times, not necessarily at the gym.

When carbs are mega-high, insulin is high, catabolism is low, anabolism is high, glycogen storage is elevated, metabolism is elevated, male hormones are 'freed,' etc., etc.
This phenomenon is what happens on high days. There isn't necessarily a direct correlation with the workout. Those carbs will be stored as glycogen and used during the workouts of the next couple of days.

Justin,

I have two questions.

1) How low would you recommend I keep my carb intake on the weekends? Would 200-300grams be low enough?

2) You also say to allow yourself to have fun on these days. What exactly do you mean by that? Would it be ok to eat a few slices of pizza? Thanks again for all the knowledge you provide!

---

1) It will vary depending on a number of factors, but that is probably a good estimate for most males.

2) Do whatever will allow you to stay on the plan. If a few slices of pizza and some beer on a Saturday allows you to be consistent the rest of the week, do it.

It's not about being perfect. No one can be perfect with their diet for the 15 years it will take to reach their ultimate goals.

But, ANYONE can be consistently GOOD for 15 years.

Justin,

I hear that it is best to gain the most muscle and least amount of fat when you start off fairly lean, around 8-10% body fat, as opposed to higher body fat levels. Is this correct? If so, would one gradually increase caloric intake for every meal upon reaching the 8-10% level to "lean-gain" as they call it?

The body is arguably most anabolic in the 10-12% body fat range.

In natural athletes, this is the body fat percentage that the body will be most efficient at producing testosterone.

As body fat levels rise, the body becomes more 'effective' at pumping out estrogen. Estrogen levels tend to rise in over fat males.

In my opinion, people worry way too much about adding weight on the scale.

Adding muscle size is a slow process even at its most efficient rate.

People want to add 30 pounds in a matter of weeks, but the vast majority of that will be fat. Then gains will likely slow down after that as the body shifts to a less anabolic state from the elevated body fat.

If you add 1 pound of pure muscle every month starting when you're 18 years old and 160 pounds, and continue adding that pound a month, every month, for 20 years, when you're 38 years old you'll be 400 pounds. And every ounce of that weight gain will be pure muscle.
You can see how unrealistic a constant progression of even one pound a month becomes over time.

I don't think people realize this when they're talking about adding 30 pounds in a few months.

A 1-pound change each month won't look like anything on the scale. You'll appear to weigh roughly the same every day. You won't even appear to weigh more from week to week. Then 6 months will pass, and you will suddenly realize you've been weighing about 5 more pounds.

Those 5 pounds every 6 months add up to huge gains as the years pass.

CONSISTENCY in gains is what most people lack.
They go crazy, trying new routines, MEGA food schedules, GORGE fests, etc., etc., and burn out after a few weeks, barely training for a while, losing weight, getting back on a "NEW" program, doing it again, etc., etc.

If that same person were to focus on eating good quality proteins, complex carbs, and essential fatty acids every 3 hours or so, every day, year round, for 15 years.....they'll be massive....without even noticing.

FOR EXAMPLE:
people love to mega dose protein, calories, junk, etc., etc.

If you were to convert JUST 10g of protein to actual new muscle protein each day (ONLY 10g out of the 100's YOU EAT), you'll gain 8 pounds of PURE muscle each year.

Muscle growth is a slow process; it is essentially immeasurable on a day-to-day basis.

So focus on being consistent with eating and training. Learn to enjoy both. Let time do the rest.

Justin,

You mentioned that during offseason training you have high carb days and normal days. Are your high carb days your training days, and off days your normal carbs? Also, as a side note, your training DVD is worth every penny.

Thanks for the comments on the DVD!

If anyone is interested, you can pick it up at www.TroponinNutrition.com

I typically take carbs somewhat higher on all training days when I'm pushing very hard. But, I generally only have 2-3 VERY high days during the week.

These days are usually over 1,000g of carbs, and are more of a job than a diet.

The extra carbs on other training days are in my pre/during/post workout shakes.

Justin,

You mentioned in one of your posts that in the offseason you have high days and normal days with carbs. Are your high days all training days? Or do you select specific days for high carb days, such as legs or back?

It depends on my motivation level, my training cycle, and my body fat.

When I'm very motivated, training hard, and my body fat is low, I'll have as many as 4 VERY high carb days per week, were I shoot for a minimum of 800g of carbs, and typically go up to 1,000g of carbs, with low fat and moderate protein.
The rest of the days are lower carb, high protein, and moderate fat.

When my motivation is lower, I'll go down to 1-2 high days per week.
To take in 1,000g of carbs, while also keeping fat low, I have to eat as frequently as every 1.5 hours.
So I'm pretty much eating rice ALL day. If I'm not motivated, I can't keep that up for long because I'll burn out.

A typical low day meal for me is:
6oz steak
1 cup white rice
1/4 cup cashews

So, roughly 60g protein, 50g carbs, and 14g added fat.

A high day meal would be:
2 scoops waxy maize with Anatrop, followed 10-20min later by:
4-6oz chicken or tilapia
2 cups white rice

This is repeated every 1.5 hours for 4 of my meals.

Justin,

First off I just want to say that I love reading your thoughts on nutrition; in particular, I enjoy your thoughts on carb cycling. For someone interested in gaining weight while limiting fat gain, how would a plan like this look? I am 190lbs and 9-11% body fat. My goal is to get to 210lbs. I lift MWF using Sheiko programs. Here's my sample nutrition plan: Monday-High Carb 350-450grams. Tuesday-Low Carb 75-125grams. Wednesday-High Carb 350-450grams. Thursday-Low Carb 75-125grams. Friday-High Carb 350-450grams. Saturday-Low Carb 75-125grams. Sunday-High Carb 350-450grams. Your thoughts and suggestions on my sample plan towards gaining weight would be greatly appreciated.

I'd do VERY high carb on training days, which would mean 3x a week. Take them around 500-600g, and be very precise with your nutrition, keeping fat intake to a minimum.
Your protein intake can be a bit lower, but still be sure to ingest around 180-200g that day.

On Tuesday, Thursday, and Friday, have low carb days.
On these days, increase your fat intake, so that you're taking in about 7-10g of healthy fats in all meals that don't have carbs. Include carbs in your first 2 meals only.

On weekends, keep carbs lower, but don't be too crazy. Allow yourself some fun on these days. This will help you be more precise during the week, which is most important on the high carb days.

On the high days, you can probably plan on taking in 150-200g of carbs in the period of time from 1 hour before your workout to 1 hour after your workout.

Justin,

What do you think is more important for muscle size, training frequency (body part per week), or training volume (sets x reps per body part)?
I'm sure you've tried both methods of training, and I am just looking for an experienced answer.

Thanks.

Nutrition.

I could be extremely brief and leave it at that...but nutrition is the most important thing for muscle size.
You cannot add muscle size without the necessary calories.
You can break it down to protein turnover, glycogen levels, positive nitrogen balance, etc., etc., but if extra protein and calories aren't available for the synthesis of new muscle, you won't grow.

Look around your gym...EVERYONE does the same exercises...there really are only a few exercises for each body part you can do.
The reason some people look like bodybuilders, some look huge, some look small, and some never grow, is food.

As for training, the most important thing is intensity. Whether you create that intensity from volume or frequency doesn't matter. If you're not training hard enough, you won't grow.

Of course...over-training is something people need to worry about...but I think that is a sham when you're beginning. It's pretty hard to get overtrained on 135lb bench presses....

I know I could bench 135lbs for a few sets every single day and not get over trained...and that is because of my food intake.
Not enough focus on nutrition is the reason almost all beginners fail in reaching their potential.

Justin,

I should have asked this question a long time ago, but better late then never. I wake up at 4 a.m. to leave for work and don't get home till about 5:15. At work (including breakfast on the way) I'll get down about 4 meals. Unfortunately, due to my lack of sleep, my metabolism has slowed down incredibly, so the stuff I used to be able to get away with, I no longer can. Even worse, due to my lack of money, (saving for college which starts in 2 weeks) and my mother's lack of willingness to support the diet, I don't have a lot of choice in my foods.

Long story short, here's the problem: I get home from the gym at about 8:30, get a protein shake in me and take a shower. Seeing as how I haven't eaten for some 5-6 hours, I know I need some food in me, but I try to get to bed by 9:30. Consequently, all the food really just sits in my stomach! I try to have as little fat and carbs as I possibly can, but sometimes my options are limited, and I know another protein shake would be a waste! What do you suggest I do/eat?!?!
Sorry for the extremely long question, but I'm trying to give you all the info I can! Thanks for your help!!

Side Note: I plan on sending in some info on me to the Great Lakes Fitness Extreme Magazine sponsorship, so look out for me. I'll be the pudgy little bird without a prayer!!

Why would another protein shake be a waste?

There's a couple of parts to this...

First, the diet...
It isn't expensive to follow the diet. I stayed on a 'good' diet in college while living in a crap apartment and having about $100 a month to buy food.

Carbs are cheap...VERY cheap.

Get a big bag of oats...old fashioned oatmeal.
Get a big bag of brown rice....a 10lb bag will last a LONG time.
If that's not enough, get a bag of taters...

Protein...more expensive.
Get eggs.
Get tuna (find the store brand...dented cans are even better...look
for the $0.39 a can special, and stock up!)
Meat....find the weekly special, and get what you can...round steak
can often be found under $2 a pound.
Protein drinks: always a cheap option.
Cottage cheese...get the big tub.

Fat:
Jug of olive oil (very cheap per serving).

I remember eating for less than $5 a day...a dozen eggs, bunch of
tuna, few protein shakes, and a ton of oatmeal. Steal the Splenda
packets from the school cafeteria when you can sneak in, or steal a
friend's meal pass card...

Second....the 5-6 hours between meals.
No excuse for that...many of us are busy. Find a way to get protein
in. Keep a protein shaker with 2-3 scoops of protein in your
car....just add water when needed.

When traveling, I've been known to eat as many as 5-6 shakes a
day and live on oatmeal cooked in the coffee pot in the hotel room.
As for metabolism...if you're eating brown rice, oatmeal, and
tuna...you aren't going to get fat...if anything, you won't be able to
eat enough to maintain weight.
When that happens, hit McD's every so often, get 4 double
cheeseburgers from the $1 menu, and double stack them into
quadruple cheeseburgers.

You're looking at 100g of protein, 100g of fat, 50g of carbs, and a
mild case of coronary ischemia for under $5...

Justin,

First I want say that I watched your DVD and you are a freakin' machine! I really enjoyed the nutritional part of the DVD; it was an eye-opener for me to actually see how a top amateur eats. I am certain you will be an IFBB Pro with that dedication in no time!

I have a few questions for you.

1) I want to eat 6 meals a day but keep missing meals (due to work, late nights in the gym, exhausted). What would you advise to fix this problem? How can I plan food intake better?

2) How do you cook your food (more specifically, what do you use? Grill, oven, etc.)? How often do you cook?

I cook all the food myself and I just collapse from exhaustion after work, gym, cooking, and then cleaning.

Any advice to help me save some time with this process would be much appreciated!

Thank you for your time Justin.

---

1) No real advice. Find a way. Consistency is the only way to reach your goals. Find a way to eat, and don't miss a meal. You won't be hungry most of the time, but eat your meals anyway.
I never leave the house if I will be gone for awhile without my meals.
I prepare my meals for the entire day each night so I am never without food.
In a bind, I always have protein powder available.
Prepare all your meals the night before, and each morning, have them set in Tupperware. Put them in a big cooler, and you will never have to worry about food.

As for work, a protein shake takes 10 seconds to slam. You are required by law to be able to take two 15-minute breaks and a 30-minute break in an 8-hour workday. There is no reason to not get the food in.

If your boss won't allow you take 10 seconds to slam a shake, report him to the Better Business Bureau.

You can even slam your shake while you're on the way to the bathroom if you have no time.

My wife and I prepare my food each night.

She throws the meat in the broiler or puts some ground beef in a big pot and lets it simmer.

We throw the rice in a rice cooker and the broccoli goes in a pot of boiling water.

When they're done, we put them in the fridge, and I measure them out into Tupperware in the morning (as you saw on the DVD).

It is difficult, and it is an extra time expense that normal people don't need to make. If it is too hard for you and not worth it, that is fine. You have to do what you enjoy in life.

I enjoy weight training and I enjoy bodybuilding. It is my choice, and the food preparation is something that is part of that.

The moment I didn't want to prepare the food or didn't want to train, I would stop.

I do this because I love it, which is really the only reason you should be doing most things in life.

Justin,

Could you make any diet suggestions for a diabetic (low carb diet) looking to gain weight?

Thank you!

I'm assuming you are a type II diabetic?

In that case, you should do quite well on a lower carb diet.

Lower carb diets will decrease the amount of insulin that your body produces, which is good, because your tissues are already desensitized to insulin.

Simple suggestions would be to focus on complex, unrefined carbohydrates.

Keep them fairly low (the amount would vary greatly depending on your size) and spread them out evenly throughout the day, with a potential dropping of carbs in your later meals.

Focus on healthy fats to replace the calories lost from lowering the carbs.

Healthy fats, especially Omega 3 fatty acids, will help increase insulin sensitivity, especially in the muscle cells, which is exactly what you want and need for proper recovery and growth from training.

A low carb diet doesn't have to be a fat loss diet.

Protein and essential fatty acids are really what fuels muscle growth. Carbohydrates decrease the amount of those nutrients you need to properly fuel growth, but those two are the real growth promoters.

Look at carbs as fuel for your training. Keep complex carbs in your diet in lower amounts, enough to fuel training, but keep them pretty low (you can probably do fine with 30g per meal).

Increase your healthy fat intake to make up the difference.

You should see your resting blood glucose levels go down quite a bit.

You are a diabetic now, but you don't have to remain a diabetic. Learn to eat correctly and teach your body to be more sensitive to insulin (by doing what I suggested), and you should be able to decrease, or even drop, your diabetic medications
(this is all assuming you're not a type I diabetic).

Justin,

I'm a type I diabetic and I know that you're really into manipulating insulin levels to obtain optimal results. What would your recommendations be for me if I'm trying to bulk up but not get too fat in the process? I know that I want to spike my insulin levels after I train, but I'm not sure by how much. I also know that you like to cycle the loads of carbs and I was just wondering if you would still recommend this for an insulin dependent diabetic. I was just recently diagnosed and I was pretty bummed at first, but the more research that I do, the more I realize that I have a potentially powerful tool if I learn how to use it optimally. Thanks for all of your help.

You have a VERY powerful tool, and one you really shouldn't be playing around with.
It is entirely different for a person with a normal functioning pancreas to try to manipulate insulin levels than it is for someone without endogenous insulin.

In case anyone is interested....in normal people, the beta cells of the islets of Langerhaans in the pancreas secrete insulin in response to blood sugar levels.
When blood sugar is elevated, the storage hormone insulin is secreted in the amount needed to transfer that blood sugar to storage areas in the body. Ideally, the blood sugar is stored as liver and muscle glycogen. Some can be converted to triglycerides and stored as fat.
Circulating protein and fatty acid levels will also be taken up and utilized more effectively.

The body is EXTREMELY efficient at taking up these nutrients on its own, and knows exactly how much insulin to secrete based on what the body's current insulin sensitivity of the tissues is.

Type II diabetes is really a decrease in sensitivity of the tissues to the presence of insulin. Just like an alcoholic won't feel the effects

from alcohol like a first time drinker would, the body can become desensitized to excessive amounts of insulin.
There are things that can increase insulin sensitivity (r-ALA, ALA, Omega 3 fatty acids, etc.)

In a type I diabetic, NO insulin is produced by the pancreas in response to blood sugar levels, and without the use of injectable insulin, the person would go into keto acidosis and could die.

You can treat the post-workout window like any other person.
A normal person will eat more carbs around his workout and HIS OWN BODY will increase insulin levels on par with the increase of blood sugar levels.

You will have to monitor and adjust this yourself.
So, you can simply take in more carbohydrates after your workout, which is what anyone would do, but it is up to you to increase your insulin dosage to keep your blood sugar at the correct level.

You may want to look into an insulin pump. You can set the bolus to the exact amount of carbs you are planning to have at any set meal, and fast-acting insulin will be timed to pump out when the carbs enter the blood stream. This is probably the most effective way that insulin dependant diabetics have to regulate blood sugar levels effectively.

Justin,

Recently I have dropped a crap load of weight. I am very strong at 225-230lbs. I am 6' and weigh 215lbs and I haven't been this cut in years. I don't want to gain too much fat but my bench press sucks at this weight. I mean, I can only bench about 350-355 raw now, as opposed to 370-375 like I used to. My deads don't suffer as much from my weight loss but man does my bench feel it. I'm taking Creatine and Omega 3 fatty acids as my supplements. Anything else you recommend taking? I eat about 4-5 times a day. Sweet potatoes, brown rice, and oatmeal as carbs sources and chicken, steak, and protein powder as protein sources. What do you recommend for gaining weight but not too much fat? Should I increase my meals to 6-8 times a day? It feels like the healthier I eat, the more I have to eat.

Thanks for your time.

Increase your meals to at least 6 times a day and go from there.

To gain weight without fat gain, try eating your normal diet 5 days a week, spreading your calories out over 6 meals, and then 2 days a week, take a HIGH carb day.
On this day, set a protein mark of around 20-30g every 2 hours, and then just pound low fat carbs as much as you can.

Keep the simple carbs to NO MORE than 50% of your carbs, preferably less, but really try to force the issue with carbs on this day.

You will be very anabolic and anti-catabolic all day from the carb intake.
Since fat intake will be extremely low on this day, you shouldn't have to worry about fat gain.
Your glycogen stores will be fully saturated after this day, which will fuel your training on your other, lower carb days.

Justin,

I just read your plan for your athletes concerning nutrition after a bodybuilding show where they eat a lot of clean food for 4 weeks and then go back to pre-contest diet for 3-4 weeks before moving on to full offseason.

I have a show in 2 weeks and am performing two 1-hour cardio sessions a day. My question is, should I stop all cardio and increase calories at the same time? It seems like this would be a huge calorie jump immediately. Is there some way to judge approximately how much to increase calories?

Also, should I jump back on my same pre-contest cardio regime during the 3-4 week mini-diet?

Thanks for your time,
Sam

Sam,
I didn't know you were doing a contest, good luck!

After the show, your hunger levels will be through the roof. Your insulin sensitivity will be sky high and your ability to store water, both intracellular and extracellular, will be sky high as well.

All these items create an environment for high levels of anabolism.

I say take advantage of it. You will be able to eat amounts of clean food that would make you vomit in the middle of the offseason.

Your insulin sensitivity will create a more likely opportunity for those nutrients to be 'placed' where you want them.

And the massive amount of water retention will provide great leverage for training.

After those 4 weeks, you may even exceed your previous offseason bodyweight high, but with less body fat than before.

At that point, your metabolism will be sky high and your ability to shed fat will be very high again.

At this point, head back into a 'pre-contest diet,' but not quite as severe (don't really need to push cardio as hard as you are now), and after 4 weeks, you will likely be VERY lean, but at a much higher weight than you were when you competed.

The first time I did this plan on myself, I went from a competition weight of around 229lbs to a peak weight of around 260-265lbs, and then back down to 245lbs after the mini-diet.

At the end of the mini-diet, I was very nearly as lean as I was at the show and 15lbs heavier.

Justin,

Just curious how you determine the amount of total calories for yourself and your clients on their high and low carb days? I have heard a good maintenance calorie guideline is to multiply your body weight by 15. What is your opinion?

You have helped me tremendously since you joined elitefts.com.

Kevin

Kevin,

I go by appearance. I'm not too big on body fat levels, calorie amounts, or anything like that.

When working with someone for a bodybuilding show, what matters is how they look so that is what I go by.

I've done this enough that I get a pretty good feel as to what a person needs by having them answer a questionnaire and send some photos.
So, I really don't even know what calorie total I recommend....

But, I used to use a guideline similar to what you posted and 15 calories per pound of bodyweight was usually a pretty good starting point.

Justin,

What would be the minimum number of lower carb days you would need? Would one do the trick? And on low days would it be cutting all carbs out and opting for veggies or just lower carbs?

Cheers!

I typically use more low carb days than high carb days.
Low carb days aren't NO carb days and they aren't 'hungry' days.
They are just a lower amount of carbohydrates replaced by a higher amount of protein and essential fats.

A high day meal may consist of something like this:
30g protein
120g carbs
no added fat

Where a low day meal may consist of something like this:
60g protein
35g carbs
15g essential fats

So, not necessarily a whole lot lower in calories, just lower in carbs.
I keep forgetting to mention this, but if anyone is interested in working with one of my nutritionists, they are less expensive than working with me and also have diet plans that are more suited to competitive bodybuilders.

Three of my nutritionists are former/current powerlifters as well. They are well versed in how to train for strength while keeping body fat where you want it, as well as maintaining strength while losing body fat.
Check them out at www.TroponinNutrition.com

Justin,

What type of diet do you recommend for someone trying to gain weight? Do you still believe that they should rotate carbs on lifting/non-lifting days or just eat as much as possible at all times?

I never believe in blindly eating as much as you can at all times to gain weight.

Each macronutrient has a specific role in supporting muscle growth. Blindly eating whatever doesn't allow you to take advantage of these roles.

I carb rotate all year.

In the offseason, I have 2-4 high carb days where the carbs are VERY high, fat is low, and protein is moderate.
The goal is to have elevated insulin levels all day.
Insulin is powerfully anti-catabolic. This allows a MUCH higher percentage of the protein you eat to be available for the synthesis of new protein.

So even though you may eat LESS protein, there is a higher *percentage* available for synthesis of new muscle tissue.

Insulin is also effective at lowering SHBG (steroid hormone binding globulin). SHBG binds to sex hormones (testosterone) and inhibits their function.
It is not the amount of testosterone in your system, but the amount of FREE testosterone, and insulin increases the potential for free testosterone in the body.

Insulin is also a storage hormone so the other macronutrients you eat are more likely to be 'stored.'

We keep fat intake minimal in an attempt to minimize fat storage.

With protein not being used for creation of new glucose and more free testosterone available in the body, we increase the likelihood that the protein we eat will be converted to new muscle tissue.

Now, insulin stores nutrients and activates glycogen synthetase to store more glycogen...but once glycogen stores are loaded up, the insulin will be looking to convert excess blood sugar to triglycerides and store them as fat....which is why we lower carbs on the non-high days to create a mildly glycogen depleted body...to allow the insulin and high carb intake to supersaturate glycogen stores.

On the low days, we increase protein intake and also raise essential fatty acid intake. This creates a caloric total that isn't necessarily much below our basal metabolic rate.

Carb intake is kept lower, but not LOW. There are still enough carbs to facilitate proper training and recovery from training. But, they are low enough to create some glycogen depletion to allow us to properly load glycogen on the high days.

With high essential and 'healthy' fatty acids, we increase the potential for sex hormone production.
Good fats and higher fat levels promote higher testosterone levels (and we increase 'free' testosterone on the high carb days).

Essential fatty acids also help fill the muscle's essential fatty acid stores and create intramuscular fat stores which can be used for energy later, and they also create a more favorable leverage environment for strength.

And of course, the protein is high to make sure we have it available for synthesis of new muscle tissue. Since carbs are lower and insulin levels will be lower, we will be more likely to use some of our dietary protein for creation of glucose to be used as energy. So, protein will be higher on this day than on the high carb days.

Justin,

I often see you writing about glycogen storage and how that occurs during your high carb days. How exactly are the carbs stored as glycogen? Why is this important?

Thanks.

Glycogen storage is a process called Glycogenesis. In this process, Glyco means glucose or glycogen, and genesis means creation. Glycogenesis is the process by which glycogen is created by adding circulating glucose molecules to glycogen.

Insulin activates the process of glycogenesis. This is yet another reason why it is important to understand the action of the insulin produced in response to the high carb intake.

Glycogenesis is actually an 11-step process.

Glycogen synthase catalyzes the 2nd step. It converts remaining glucose one by one into glycogen chains.

Glycogen synthase is activated by phosphoprotein phosphatase.

Phosphoprotein phosphatase is activated by insulin. In layman's terms: Insulin activates phosphoprotein phosphatase, which activates glycogen storage.

This is important because the glycogen we store on high carb days will be available for use as fuel on the lower carb days. This allows us to maintain a sufficient energy source to fuel workouts, while also keeping calories and insulin lower to fight fat storage. On low and medium carb days, our protein and essential fatty acid intake will be higher, but thanks to the glycogenesis from high days, we still have an abundance of energy for use.

Justin,

I've been reading your log and Q&A on elitefts.com and just wondered if you could do the opposite with your current carb cycling to help trick the metabolism for weight gain. So have mostly high carb days and then maybe one or two low carb days so the body doesn't adjust? Have you ever done anything like this?

Thanks.

I do that in the offseason.
I have as many as 4 very high days in the offseason, with all the other days being "lower" carb days with higher levels of essential fatty acids.
I find it allows me to continually progress, maintain a relatively low body fat level, and keep my insulin sensitivity high.

Justin,

When trying to gain muscle, what do you think of supplements like r-ALA for your very high carb days?

---

r-ALA has some benefits.
Besides being a good antioxidant, it should help the body utilize the carbohydrates you ingest, as well as help maintain a higher level of insulin sensitivity for all days of the week.

I recommend it quite frequently to my clients.

Justin,

Thanks for your response to my question about post-contest nutrition.

I have a follow-up question about your carb cycling protocol that you posted in your training log. For your cheat meal listed on the Saturday low day, do you go crazy for one meal, or do you just get a little of the food you've been craving without overdoing it?

I want to add a Saturday cheat meal to my carb cycling schedule (because it is my offseason) but am concerned that I will do some serious damage. It's nothing for me to eat an entire large pizza by myself in one sitting and follow it up with half a box of cookies or a large ice cream.

Do you have any thoughts on this?

My cheat meal this past Saturday was the following:
12 buffalo wings
side order of fries
1/2lb black and bleu burger
chicken, bacon, and ranch wrap with chips and salsa
Corona
Fudge cake dessert with ice cream
So....it was a full-on cheat.

I will tame these meals and eventually eliminate them as I get closer to the show.

But, if I'm having a cheat meal, I'm eating...I don't want to spend the next week wishing I would have enjoyed the only time I had a chance to enjoy the food.

A cheat meal is a shock to the body. It will elevate metabolism and teach the body that calories and nutrients are in abundance so there is no reason to attempt to horde nutrients (store fat...) for later needs.

Justin,

I have been reading your posts about nutrition and dieting and I had a couple of questions:

1) What is the basic idea behind the low carb/high protein day followed by a high carb/low protein day?

2) Could someone benefit from doing a day where they eat 2 grams of carbs and 1 gram of protein per lbm (high carb day) and then the next day 1 gram carbs/2 grams of protein per lbm (high protein day)?

Thanks for your time and answers.

Matt

---

1) The reasons for carb and calorie rotating are various. You have a limited capacity to store glycogen. When in an offseason mode, your glycogen stores are typically close to being 'full.'
In this case, continuous ingestion of carbohydrates at a high level can create an environment for fat gain.
By lowering carbohydrate amount without drastically lowering calorie amount, you can create an iso-caloric diet where you become mildly depleted of glycogen stores.
This allows you to more effectively store glycogen on high carb days.

Periods of mild glycogen depletion and lower carbohydrate meal plans can increases insulin sensitivity as well. This will aid in your assimilation of the carbohydrates on high days.
When dieting, your body will attempt to adapt to any caloric level. When you follow an iso-caloric diet day after day, your body learns to set that caloric amount as its resting metabolic rate. This can happen no matter how low your calories are. So, in order to continue fat burning, you must lower calories even further, until your body's resting metabolic rate is slowed to that level

eventually.

With carb rotation, you attempt to create a situation where the "high" day is your metabolic rate.

By ingesting calories and carbohydrates at a high level, the body realizes that food is plentiful, and it doesn't need to slow down its metabolism.

The high day also re-saturates glycogen stores, which you can then feed on to fuel training and other energy needs on low carb days without needing to utilize as much protein for the conversion to glucose.

2) People could certainly benefit from the approach you gave.

I vary my carbohydrate amounts year-round. I feel it allows me to stay lean, stay strong, and never have to go to extremes to lose or gain size and/or body fat.

Justin,

I just competed in my first bodybuilding show this past weekend, placing 3rd in the light heavy class. My contest weight was 195. After a few days of eating pretty good, I am ready to go back to an offseason type diet. I want to maintain a quality physique and stay around 10-12% body fat. I think this would mean my weight should be around 215-220. Do you have any input or suggestions concerning the offseason? I guess I'm looking for some tips on how to stay relatively lean but still add some quality muscle.

Thanks in advance for your input.

I like to have people go right into offseason mode after a contest.

Your insulin sensitivity is high, your hunger is through the roof, and your ability to assimilate nutrients is about as high as it is going to get.

So, for about 4 weeks after a show, I have people eat a full-on offseason diet. My offseason diets are all good, clean calories, so it isn't a "bulk" diet at all. I really don't like that term to be quite honest.

Then after 4 weeks of that, we go into a diet for 3-4 weeks, which is pretty similar to a pre-contest diet in terms of strictness.

At the end of those 4 weeks, you will be very nearly as lean as you were at the show, but should be MUCH heavier.

At this time, I take a break from training (usually a maximum of 2-3 days for me, as I just can't stay away from the gym, especially when I can eat well), and begin my "real" offseason prep.

My offseason prep starts with me being quite lean, larger than I was at my show, and with my body in a state where it is ready to assimilate nutrients efficiently.

I believe I make the majority of my gains in any given year in this period after my show.

For the most part, my bodyweight climbs higher than my previous offseason high within 4 weeks of my show, and after the diet, I'm still pretty heavy, although quite lean.

It is tough to go back into something so regimented after a long diet, but I feel it is worth it.

Justin,

1) What type of caloric intake do you think I should shoot for, given these parameters?
Current: 27 y/o, 5'10", 170 lbs., 12-13% body fat, 265 BN, 345 SQ, 405 DL
Goal: 180 lbs., Under 10% body fat, Bigger lifts across the board

2) Should I eat more or less (or a different carb/protein mix) on the days that I do not train or just keep it consistent every day? I lift 3-4 times per week almost always after 7 p.m. (Joe D's WS4SB program).

I always eat fewer calories, and especially fewer carbohydrates, on days I don't train. I would recommend the same to anyone.

Training is a much bigger calorie burner than most people expect.

I really go by photos more than by weight when designing plans, but I would guess that you would want to shoot for roughly 1.5g of protein per lb of LBM on high carb days, with up to 2g of carbs, and around 2g of protein per lb of LBM on med and low carb days, with carbs dropping as low as .25g per lb of LBM at your lowest.

Bring the big calories and carbs in around your training sessions, and don't be scared to be a bit hungry on off days. By being mildly glycogen depleted going into high days, you will create an environment for more efficient glycogen storage on the high days.

Justin,

1) How do you feel about milk as a nutritional tool?

2) With mass gaining, can you really drink too much of it?

---

1) I'm not a huge fan of milk really. I rarely drink it at any point in the year.
Milk protein is a complete protein, so it is certainly not a useless source of nutrients.
But the carbohydrate mix in milk is a mix I'm not a major fan of.

The lactose in milk is a disaccharide, consisting of glucose and galactose.

While it doesn't hold true to as high of a level in America, as much as 70% of the world is lactose intolerant. So right off the bat, this poses a problem with milk.

If you're not lactose intolerant, the milk sugar isn't a superior carbohydrate source for a consistent energy source in a hard training individual.

I'm not 100% opposed to milk. If I have cereal, I have milk. I love the taste of milk, in all forms from skim to whole, but because it doesn't fit perfectly into "my" nutritional program, I don't drink a ton of it.

2) I am not a fan of mass gaining at all. I am a fan 100% of gaining muscle mass as quickly as possible. But gaining mass by adding size (body fat, water, and muscle) as quickly as possible is unhealthy and not the most effective means of progress, in my opinion.

Most studies on the subject show that we are most anabolic (in terms of hormonal production and nutrient digestion and assimilation) at around 10-12% body fat, which is actually a fairly low body fat percentage.

As we gain body fat, our bodies actually become LESS efficient at gaining muscle and MORE efficient at storing body fat.

Higher body fat levels have been associated with higher estrogen levels.
Higher body fat levels lower insulin sensitivity in muscle tissue and the argument can be made that it increases insulin sensitivity in adipose tissue....so, your body learns to NOT bring nutrients to the muscle but becomes BETTER at storing them as fat.

Justin,

Thanks for all the great nutritional info....but I have a question about nutrition for the "Average Joe's" out there like myself.

I work a professional job about 50 hours a week and I get to the gym about 3-4 nights per week for 1 to 1.5 hours.

I follow Joe D's WS4SB template. I mostly lift weights, with minimal cardio. My metabolism is naturally pretty high. I'm 27 y/o 5'10" 170 lbs. with approx 13% body fat. My max bench is 265 lbs. My max squat is 345 lbs. My max DL is 405 lbs.

I'm not trying to win any contests, just looking to get to about 180 lbs and 10% body fat while maintaining my speed and athleticism, without compromising health.

I'm not interested in supplements (other than a post-workout shake) or fat burners, and I can't see myself working out more frequently than I currently do, although I am INTENSE during the times that I do workout.

I imagine there are a whole lot more of my type out there than the more advanced guys like yourself and the other EFS guys who work in the industry.
Considering the info that I gave you, what type of nutritional plan would you put me on?

I appreciate any info you can provide.

Thanks,
Bryan

I would put you on the same plan as anyone else.
Nutrition really shouldn't be a time consuming thing.

I work a full time job, own and run www.TroponinNutrition.com, work with www.TrueProtein.com, and my wife and I do all our own shipping of supplements and DVDs. I can definitely sympathize with the long work hours and minimal time.

But, for me, it is easier to eat the way I do than eat normally.

I prepare all my food at night; it takes about 20 minutes total. I throw my meat in the oven broiler (mine fits 4lbs of meat typically), put all my rice in a pot, and my broccoli in another pot.

When it is all done, I divide it up into my meals (I often do this in the morning).
My wife and I do it while we are cleaning up the kitchen, doing dishes, etc.

I eat my meals when I can throughout the day.
A meal may be timed for 3 p.m.....and I may take a few bites then, a few more 20 minutes later, and I may not finish until after 4pm...but I get the meals in.

Once you get into the 'groove' of preparing food, you'll find that you spend less time preparing your food than if you would just hit the drive-thru (which can take 20 minutes for one meal at some of the places near me...).

GENERAL NUTRITION

Justin,

I always hear the term "protein synthesis." I understand that this is how we build muscle, but how does this happen? Does our body just take the protein from our food and attach it to the muscle tissue?

Thanks.

Protein synthesis is the process by which cells build proteins. This process involves transcription and translation, which cannot accurately be covered in brief.

Protein synthesis can roughly be explained as the process by which proteins are created from amino acids.

Just as proteins are created by protein synthesis, amino acids are created from amino acid synthesis.

Amino acid synthesis is the process by which amino acids are produced from other compounds. Humans are only capable of producing 12 of the 20 amino acids needed for protein synthesis. The other 8 amino acids must be included in the diet.

These amino acids are called the Essential Amino Acids.

Essential Amino Acids:
  Isoleucine

Leucine
Lysine
Threonine
Tryptophan
Methionine
Valine
Phenylalanine

A 9th amino acid, Histidine, is technically considered an essential amino acid, although it is mostly only infants and children who cannot properly synthesize it.

There are also other amino acids that are considered "Conditionally Essential Amino Acids," as they are not able to be created in sufficient quantities under various circumstances. Glutamine is an example of this.

Each amino acid plays crucial roles in many processes of the body.

What is most important to remember is that all the essential amino acids must be present in the diet and all 20 amino acids must be present at the site of protein synthesis for synthesis to occur.

This is called the "all or none principle."

In protein synthesis, since all amino acids must be present at the site of synthesis, the amino acid in the lowest quantity then becomes the limiting amino acid.

Complete proteins are foods that contain all the essential amino acids in the food. Meat sources, including milk and eggs, are complete proteins.
Many plant sources are incomplete protein sources, meaning they lack one or more of the essential amino acids.

So, to re-cap, all the essential amino acids must be included in the diet for protein synthesis to occur. The protein of lowest concentration will then become the limiting protein in protein synthesis.

You can see why meat, eggs, protein powders, and other bodybuilding staples are so important to muscle growth. These sources are complete proteins, including all the essential amino acids, and since they're muscle tissue of other animals, there is no major deficiency in any one protein. This prevents a limiting protein of any major significance.

Justin,

I was told that there may be mercury in fish and fish oil. I take a fish oil supplement most days. Should I cut this out of my routine? Is it dangerous to take fish oil? I know how big of a risk aspartame is, and don't want to add another danger to my diet.

People involved with weight training tend to overdo everything.

To prevent deficiencies, you need a rather small amount of Omega 3 fatty acids.

What is arguably more important is the *ratio* of Omega 3, 6, and 9.

Americans tend to be very deficient in Omega 3 fatty acids comparatively.

But we need to keep things in perspective.
The obesity epidemic is killing Americans. 50% of us are going to die of heart disease.

Low levels of Omega 3 fatty acids can aid in lowered insulin sensitivity....leading to diabetes, which leads to heart disease....which is going to KILL 1/2 of everyone in America (as stated above).

I'll pick my poison. Everything has risks.

I'll worry more about the American diet killing 50% of us through heart disease than 'possible' problems from taking something that Americans are grossly deficient in and helps heart disease, which is our greatest risk.

Justin,

Thanks for your help with my past questions.

I'm just wondering how you cook your eggs. I like them scrambled with a bit of olive oil, but would that "denature" the amino acids?

Thanks again.

It probably won't denature them enough to make a huge difference.

It will reduce the chance of salmonella poisoning though.

Humans have been cooking meat for quite some time. If it caused enough denaturing to have a major effect, we wouldn't have survived.

Justin,

I have been eating brown rice for a long time and noticed you eat white rice. I was always told that white rice was "bad" for you. Is one better than the other? Sorry if it seems like I am splitting hairs.

Thank you for your time,
Will

They're the same food.

White rice has the outer 'husk' removed via a milling process. Milling is often called 'whitening' for this reason.

The outer shell gives it the brown color, and is essentially all a fibrous mass. This lowers the GI of the rice, as the husk doesn't allow as rapid of an uptake into the blood stream.

White rice has the outer portion removed. This causes a quicker uptake into the bloodstream, resulting in a higher insulin spike. The removal of the outer layer will also lower fiber and mineral content.

1 cup of cooked white rice is about 50g of carbs.
1 cup of cooked brown rice is about 35g of carbs.

So, they're the same carb, but the white rice just has the fibrous outer layer taken off.

I have a hard time taking in enough calories when I eat brown rice, so I use the more calorie-dense white rice when needed.

Justin,

This is a really stupid question. But it will solve a bet. Do you ever completely mess up cooking and just eat it anyway? I mean overcook, undercook, etc.

If the meat is still chewy in the middle, I'll just nuke it really good when I re-heat it at work.

If the meat is really tough, I just pretend it is beef jerky.

I've left chicken in the oven for a few hours more than once.

As a general rule, the longer a protein is exposed to heat, and the higher the heat, the more the protein gets denatured.
So, all things being equal, overcooking is probably worse than undercooking for protein absorption (but better for bacteria levels).

Over the course of a 20-year career, a few overcooked meals probably aren't going to make a huge difference.

Justin,

This is probably a stupid question. I'm a college student and I don't usually get out of bed until around 12 in the afternoon. I was always under the impression that you had to start your eating earlier in the morning. This won't affect my diet, will it?

The day has 24 hours. People typically sleep 6-8 of those. (College kids might get to sleep a bit more).
Whether you get up at 6 a.m. or noon, you generally still have the same number of waking hours and the same amount of time to get your meals in.
Your eating day will start later, but will end later too, to coincide with your wake/sleep schedule.

Justin,

Is it necessary to use whey if you get enough protein from food? My budget is tight and I figured that I would spend the money on just creatine and beta-alanine instead.

It is only necessary to get all essential amino acids in your diet and enough total protein to prevent a deficiency in any particular amino acid (the limiting amino acid).

Other than that, there are no real necessities for sustaining life.

Whey is really just a rapidly-digesting complete protein with a good amino acid profile.
It has its benefits, especially in times when rapid uptake of amino acids is beneficial, but it's not entirely necessary.

Whey prices are skyrocketing right now and companies are going to be coming out with some cool new products very soon.

It's a tough time for supplement companies because the price of whey is climbing.
But it's an exciting time too, because the smart companies will use this as an opportunity to come out with BETTER forms of protein.

Justin,

I've just read your article, "High Molecular Weight Carbohydrates." I was wondering if there are any foods that contain this kind of thing, or do I have to buy the drink itself? If there aren't, are there any foods that are high in dextrose?

Thank you for your time.

Dextrose is dirt cheap.
Dextrose is just glucose. Glucose is a sugar. It is actually D-glucose, named for its dextro-rotary appearance when looking at it with a light microscope.
So, you get dextro-rotary glucose...or dextrose.

Waxy maize is a specific type of corn starch processed in a particular way. You won't find that specific food in isolation in any 'normal' food.

Dextrose is not very costly to purchase and can be found at most bulk nutrition centers.

Waxy maize is more expensive. In my opinion, it is worth the extra cost.

If you're absolutely set against ingesting food in shake form, any food high in carbohydrates and protein will benefit you post-workout.

Justin,

I have seen your pre/during/post-workout protocol and I was wondering how I should tweak it? I am a newbie powerlifter, following the Westside Beginners Manual program. My primary goal is to get strong. I am more concerned with getting strong for my body weight than being super huge. Body weight currently is 203lbs.

Thanks a lot for the help.

If you're trying to keep your body weight down and are around 200lbs, I would suggest the following:

Limit the bulk of your carb intake to meal 1, or meal 1 and 2 (i.e. early in the day).

Then, follow this protocol around your workout:
BEFORE TRAINING: 1 scoop Anatrop, 50g waxy maize
DURING TRAINING: 1 scoop Anatrop, 35g waxy maize
POST TRAINING: 1 scoop Anatrop, 1 scoop whey isolate, 50g waxy maize.

Have a normal meal about 1 hour after your post-workout shake.

This will create the best environment for high availability of creatine, essential amino acids, and blood glucose during your training. It will also create an environment for high levels of water inside the muscle cell, which will create beneficial leverages for lifting. It will also make certain you have all the proven essential nutrients available to stimulate protein synthesis and to aid in recovery after the workout.

You can get Anatrop at www.TroponinNutrition.com,
Waxy maize at: www.trueprotein.com,
and everything else at www.elitefts.com.

Make sure you mix the mixture with a sugar-free drink like Crystal Light, as the amino acids in the Anatrop have a 'bite.' The high levels of L-leucine in Anatrop create a bitter taste. Even though it is flavored, I like to mix it with another light flavoring.

It is also important to add as much water as possible. The more water you use, the more effective the waxy maize will be.

Justin,

Would eating breakfast last thing in the morning, let's say 10 o'clock, be hindering muscle gains? And also, is high salt or low salt in the diet best for strength? Why?

Thanks for your time.

What do you mean by eating breakfast last thing in the morning?

If you mean after you've done the triple S (shit, shower, shave...) and dressed yourself (and any children requiring assistance), then there is a simple answer.

That answer is....ahh...probably...no...possibly...or maybe not...depends on a few factors...and how long of a time frame...and...well...

All things being equal, if you're in a negative nitrogen balance and in an energy deficit in the morning from fasting all night, your growth potential will be lower than if you ingested growth-promoting nutrients immediately upon rising, or better yet, never allowed your blood amino pools to drop into a state of negative nitrogen balance.

But, all things aren't always equal.
As long as you don't wait forever to eat, you should be fine.

A high salt diet will create an environment for elevated intracellular and extracellular water levels. This will decrease over time somewhat, as aldosterone levels adapt to the high sodium diet. But higher levels of water retention in the body can create better leverages across the joints.
So, while a high sodium diet may not be as healthy, it is likely better for strength...due to the increased leverage abilities at the joints.

Justin,

Is the saturated fat found in meats, cheeses, etc. any unhealthier than the saturated fat found in nuts, oats, and other plant products? Obviously there's more of it in animal-derived foods but is plant saturated fat any healthier than animal saturated fat? Saturated fat for us carnivores is something that's very easy to overdo it seems.

Thanks.

The body needs a mix of Omega 3, 6, and 9 fatty acids.

Omega 3 fatty acids are found in fish, nuts, and other 'good' things. This is the anti-inflammatory fat. Americans are typically lacking in this.

Omega 6 fatty acids are found in many sources as well, including most foods Americans tend to eat.
These are more inflammatory. One of the things Omega 6 fats break down to is arachidonic acid. Arachidonic acid is one of the most potent growth regulators of the human body. Some supplements out right now take advantage of arachidonic acid's benefits.
Another Omega 6 fat is Gamma Linolenic acid (GLA). I recently wrote an article on GLA for EliteFTS. GLA has many fat-burning benefits and has been linked to many levels of obesity when it is deficient in the diet. GLA is actually a fat that burns fat.

Omega 9 fatty acids aren't actually essential, as the body can create them from other fatty acids, but we typically get a decent amount of Omega 9's in the American diet anyway.
They are typically found in things like olive oil.

Saturated fats are found in abundance in American diets and it is very unlikely that any American is lacking in saturated fat intake. There are different types of saturated fats though. The saturated

fats found in meats are longer chains of fat...something like 16-18 carbons typically.
Butter is a short-chain saturated fat and some oils like coconut oil are medium-chain saturated fats.

The length of the chain does have some effects in how the body processes the fat. But...in my opinion, you don't need to worry about the differences in saturated fat between various sources. Just try to minimize it and make sure you're getting plenty of healthy essential fatty acids from nuts, fish, and other 'good' junk.

Justin,

Two questions:
1) Do you think it is important to lower protein intake every now and then? I've heard (and question) that the body becomes accustomed to it and begins using it as fuel instead of for building muscle.
2) How important do you think it is to change exercises? Looking though some of the logs on EliteFTS and what people typically recommend, I see the same basic exercises with maybe some change in rep, set, or order. When I do see change, it's usually short term or for another staple exercise, like dumbbell presses for bench presses.

---

1) If the body is in an anabolic state and synthesis of new muscle is a priority, the body will utilize protein.
There are only 3 macronutrients and only 2 of them are essential. The only two nutrients the body needs to sustain life (besides water) are protein and fat.
That is ALL the body has to sustain life. I just don't see how the body would/could choose to become desensitized to one of those. There is no major effect on blood sugar to create a chance at decreased insulin sensitivity of the tissues as there is with carbohydrates. So there is no real benefit for the body to become 'accustomed' to protein.

The body does what is best to sustain life; that's really all it is. And I don't see how desensitivity to protein increases the likelihood for survival in any way.

If a need to synthesize new muscle tissue from protein is present, the body will utilize available protein for that.
If the need is not present, the protein will be converted to glucose, used as energy, stored as glycogen, or eventually converted to triglycerides and potentially stored as fat....same as it always was.

2) You see the top guys using the same exercises...it is because that is what works.

I don't buy into the need to change exercises all the time.

The basic exercises involve the most muscle groups and create the most potential for muscle trauma to later be repaired into larger and stronger muscle fiber.

If my body becomes 'used' to squatting...I'm not going to be convinced that switching to leg extensions is going to increase my leg size.

I see lots of guys at the gym using the pec deck...so many that the machine is never open!
I see lots of guys doing hyperextensions and pulldowns...

I see very few doing deadlifts and squats...but those are the guys who I would rather look like.

Justin,

How do you typically cook your chicken/steak? Do you use an outdoor grill or Foreman? Any seasonings or marinades? What's your thought on white rice pre-contest? Always appreciated!

Thanks again!

I prefer to grill my steak and I like to poach my chicken...I think that's what it's called.

I cut up the chicken into little chunks. I coat a pan with soy sauce (not a pot, but a fairly deep/big pan) and then put the chicken in. I pour water into the pan until it covers the chicken. Then I add various seasonings.
I let it cook on med/high heat until the water boils off and the chicken is left...very moist.

I use a TON of seasoning. I'm a salt freak.
Lawrys, garlic salt, salt, sea salt… hell, anything with sodium.

I don't use many marinades because I don't have much time. If I have time to marinate the meat, I probably won't have time to cook it later...I have to get it done when the time is available.

I'm not against white rice pre-contest, but it is so much more calorie-dense than brown rice. I'd rather eat 2 cups of brown rice than just over a cup of white rice....makes me feel fuller.

Justin,

Thank you very much for the nutritional advice. I am a type II diabetic. Are there any supplements you'd recommend for my situation?

Stay strong!

There are many 'insulin potentiators' that claim to be effective for people in your situation.

Chromium: In the 50's (I think), there were patients being fed intravenously who were showing signs of being diabetics even though they weren't. Chromium was known to be involved in the body's response to insulin. When chromium was added to the IV feedings, the patient's blood sugar returned to normal.
So chromium (sold as chromium picolinate) is necessary for the body to properly utilize the effects of insulin.
I doubt this is needed...we get plenty in our diet.

r-ALA or ALA: Can lower blood sugar levels by increasing insulin sensitivity. By making the cells of the body more sensitive to insulin, the body can produce less insulin in response to carb ingestion but still maintain normal blood sugar levels.
This makes the insulin you DO produce more effective in the cells while keeping insulin production lower to help keep its fat storing effects at bay.
I do believe this will help diabetics, as it essentially mimics the way most oral diabetic meds work.

I have seen studies showing diabetics lowering doses or even dropping their diabetic medications after supplementing with r-ALA or ALA.

Omega 3 fatty acids: Omega 3 fatty acids have many benefits in the body. One of them is increasing the sensitivity of cells to insulin....a DECREASE in insulin sensitivity is essentially what diabetes is. Omega 3's have also shown (at least in some studies) to be more specific to muscle cell insulin sensitivity, which is exactly what we want as weight trainers.

Cinnamon: Has shown to increase insulin sensitivity as well and is often touted as a weight loss aid. Works in a similar manner to the others I've listed.

Vanadyl Sulfate: Was touted highly in the 80's and 90's as a replacement for insulin. Probably not all it was cracked up to be, but some studies have shown vanadyl to increase insulin sensitivity and make your insulin more effective, thus lowering blood sugar. Many of the studies have extraneous factors that may have skewed the results though.

There are more out there as well. Some products will even have all these ingredients in them.

I would recommend supplementing with Omega 3 fatty acids at each meal, even if it is a few grams.
Also, try r-ALA at a dose of 100-300mg or more each day. You can try taking 100-200mg with breakfast and post- workout.

If you use ALA, you will need a higher dose, roughly 600mg per dose.

Also, make sure you're eating complex carbohydrates, plenty of fiber, healthy fats, and avoiding sugar. Most diabetics would be able to control their diabetes fairly well with just diet modifications.

Exercise is almost like a dose of insulin and one of the best things a diabetic can do to lower blood sugar levels naturally. Make sure you're doing some form of exercise each day, even if it is pretty low intensity some of the days.

A simple walk in the morning can go a long way in controlling blood sugar for the day.

Justin,

How did you go about learning everything you know about nutrition? I really want to learn as much as I can about nutrition.

When I was 14 or 15, I started getting into working out and changing the way I looked. For whatever reason, the nutrition aspect of all that intrigued me.
So, I began asking for nutrition books for birthdays and Christmas, etc.

Eventually, when I went to college, I majored in Exercise Science, which was pretty much 4 years of anatomy, physiology, and nutrition.
That was a good starting point.

I still read things all the time and am always on Pub Med, Google, even Wikipedia, looking up or going back over things.

I'm a brief-package-of-information junkie, so Wikipedia, magazines, Pub Med, etc., are great for me.

I always tell people to get a college physiology or nutrition textbook and go from there. If you understand the background of nutrition and digestion, it will make understanding all the little things much easier.

Justin,

I like to put a lot of my vegetables and fruits in a blender because it's easier for me to ingest them and I just don't taste certain foods when they are blended with others. With that being said, how do you feel about doing this? I'm asking because I've read that the ingestion of certain things can mess with the absorption of others. For example, calcium may blunt the absorption of zinc. Should I avoid putting dairy products such as milk, cottage cheese, and yogurt in my shakes if I mix them with broccoli? (I know this sounds nasty but I'll blend anything) If so, any other foods you'd recommend not mixing?

You shouldn't have to worry much about foods 'blocking' the absorption of another nutrient.
You may not maximally absorb each particular nutrient when foods are eaten, but the human body is pretty efficient at uptake and utilization of necessary nutrients.

We wouldn't have survived thousands of years of struggling to find enough nutrition for survival if this was the case.

In today's society, vitamin and mineral deficiencies aren't a major cause for concern.

Justin,

How do you feel about all this talk saying fruits and vegetables today do not contain as many vitamins and such as they did 50 or so years ago? Do you feel this is a problem to be considered?

They probably do not contain as many vitamins and minerals as 50 years ago, and 50 years ago possibly didn't contain as much as 5,000 years ago.

Today's methods of farming produce larger and more plentiful crops of fruits and vegetables.

When a fruit grows larger, the taste is not necessarily better...and it is not necessarily as nutritious. The extra 'size' of the fruit will be mostly water, which will actually decrease the level of sugar (sweetness) in the fruit, and will decrease the relative quantity of vitamins and minerals.
But, bigger fruits sell better...

Vegetable crops today can be much more compact than previously.

Fertilizer usage is much more effective, which allows more vegetable per square foot than years ago.
This could potentially decrease the amount of vitamins and minerals that each particular vegetable has.

But vitamin and mineral deficiencies are VERY unlikely in today's society.

We are dealing with an entirely different problem today.

Malnutrition has been almost completely erased in developed countries and replaced with obesity and 'over nutrition.'

There just isn't a lack of nutrients in most people's diets. If there is a chance that we might be lacking in any nutrient, we will cram that nutrient into a new "vitamin-fortified" food.

Justin,

We all know we love a nice six-pack on the weekend, especially in the summer time during a nice barbecue. Here is the question: What do you guys feel is the healthiest option while consuming beer? I myself prefer Michelob Ultra. Are there any others that match up?

Thanks and keep up the good work,

JC

The problem with beer isn't really the carbs. It's the alcohol... Alcohol has about 7 calories per gram, whereas carbs have roughly 4 calories per gram.

So if you have a low-carb beer, you're saving yourself a few grams of carbs per beer....but that is kind of a drop in the bucket compared to the high amount of empty calories (the alcohol) you're taking in.

All things being equal, Michelob Ultra, or another low carb source is probably better....but if I'm drinking beer....I'm drinking the good stuff until I can't taste it anymore, then I'm drinking the cheap stuff until I can't focus anymore.

After that, I'm probably looking for some liquor in the back of the freezer, talking very loudly back and forth with another drunk friend about something that happened 10 years ago that we've now turned into pure hyperbole....or not noticing that my 'witty jokes' aren't hitting quite the level of funny that I think they are...things of that nature.

Justin,

Would you guys recommend eating more fish rather than taking fish oil?

I don't think you'll find a huge difference either way.

While fish oils capsules may seem less 'natural,' they are taken from the same source as eating the fish....from the fish themselves.

Eating fish is usually a good idea. Most American diets are lacking in fish for sure.

With my diets, I prefer to use fish capsules in conjunction with eating fish, as it allows me to better control the amount of fish oil and Omega 3's I take in while still getting them directly from the source.

Justin,

What are some of the ways of supporting an athlete's adrenal support? When someone is burned out and sluggish, what do you offer or what is a protocol that could be followed?

Thanks.
Steve

I don't have a particular method of adrenal support for people who are burned out besides limiting stimulants.

Many people, in my opinion, rely too heavily on stimulants for training, and especially dieting.

I've fallen into that trap myself. Life is busy, and it is hard to be motivated for training when there is so much else to do.

But continued over-stimulation of the adrenal glands from taking stimulants is going to create a backlash at some point.

I believe it is a major contributor to the extreme fatigue, sluggishness, and water weight gain many bodybuilders experience after a long contest diet where stimulants are taken in abundance.

Caffeine will create "withdrawals" when discontinued. So you will want to slowly taper off that.

I think you'll find that once you've taught your body to function at a high level without the stimulants, you will feel much better and potentially grow much better.

I used no stimulants in 2005/2006, and made the best gains of my life.

Remember that stimulation of the CNS is activating the 'fight or flight' response in the body. And in that situation, the body is NOT concerned with synthesizing new muscle or sparing muscle tissue from energy use. It is concerned with utilizing whatever means are necessary to get you out of the situation...which can easily include using muscle tissue for energy.

Unfortunately, I let myself get back into the mode of pre-workout caffeine use this past year, out of feeling fatigued from being so busy....mild usage gradually turned into caffeine use before all workouts by the end of the offseason.

I honestly feel like I negated some potential for gains I could have had otherwise.

Justin,

I'd like to get your opinion on 2 things:
1) What do you think about putting raw eggs into
shakes....good or bad idea?
2) Do you think fasting is ever necessary?
Thanks for all the info. I saw some of your videos on
YouTube.... pretty impressive. Keep up the good work.

1) There is probably little risk to adding the raw eggs. Raw eggs can deplete your biotin stores however, and biotin is an important nutrient in energy balance in the body. If you do this regularly, be sure to supplement with a B-complex vitamin.

2) Unfortunately, or fortunately, depending on how you look at it, I'm not really in the practice of "health." My nutritional advice is geared towards performance and appearance.

I don't personally believe that fasting improves performance or appearance, so I'm not a big fan of it.

Justin,

Hey, how important do you think it is to get food in the body
right after waking up? I always eat a good breakfast in the
a.m. but sometimes it's a half hour to hour after I actually
wake up. Should I down some BCAA's or a protein shake right
when I wake up?

I really don't stress about it all that much.
You do want to get nutrients in, especially protein in the morning, but in my opinion it isn't a huge deal if you wait 30 minutes.

In all reality, stressing about not eating is probably doing way more damage than not eating.

Justin,

What do you think about low carb milk? Is it any more worthwhile than regular milk? I'd imagine that the protein would remain the same and the carbs would be limited, but I really have no idea. What are your thoughts?

If I remember from looking at the labels, the protein is actually higher than regular milk.

I think it is a good product for those wishing to keep carbohydrates lower while enjoying the taste of milk.

It is going to be more processed than regular milk, which may or may not affect the "health" of the product.

I used to get one brand of the milk fairly regularly a few years ago. I haven't bought it in a long time though...not sure why.

The chocolate version tasted like melted ice cream. I remember it being a very good taste when waking up in the middle of the night.

Justin,

I coach high school girl's track. I was wondering what would be a good diet for our sprinters and distance runners. The basics don't seem to be working well enough. All the girls are multi-event competitors. We have meets twice a week. Though we are doing very well, I have found one of our distance girls a bit dehydrated and some sprinters running out of gas.

Thanks.

If their diets are like most HS kids' diets, I can imagine why.

First of all, make sure they're staying hydrated.
DO NOT restrict water or water breaks during practice. I don't think this is in practice much anymore, but it used to be in "style" for coaches to restrict water during practice to make kids "tougher."

This is incredibly counter-productive and does nothing but get less performance out of the kids and risk health problems.

If you have Gatorade available at meets, encourage kids to create a 50/50 Gatorade/water mix.
This is arguably better than full-strength Gatorade at keeping hydration levels up and blood glucose levels steady.
Also, continue to stress the importance of proper nutrition before meets.
Let the competitors know that if they are lacking in fuel, they will not compete to the best of their abilities.

You can keep it simple and recommend some basic food sources. It will be better for them to eat oatmeal with some healthy fats and lean protein sources before the meets instead of a Pop Tart and some candy on the way to school...but good luck getting a 17 year-old kid to cook that....and good luck getting the average American family to eat that meal with him...

A simple suggestion would be for the kids to have some kind of red sauce pasta the night before (basically spaghetti).
The white flour noodles may not be the greatest choice, but it is simple for them to remember, and if it is meat-based as well, it will provide all they need for fuel.

In the morning, try to get them to eat a good breakfast. Something that is a decent carb source is actually Cheerios...they are made from oats, and when mixed with skim milk, are a good source of fiber, complex carbs, and protein.

Also make sure they're eating during the meets. Most kids know to bring things like oranges, which are good, but they generally lack in calories for a long day.

Something simple, such as telling them to pack a turkey or tuna sandwich, bananas, and plenty to drink....or even suggesting they go to Subway and get a whole wheat sub, will provide them with a better mix of calories and nutrients to fuel the meet.

It is hard to get kids to eat correctly and going at them full bore with top level nutrition is probably going to put them off.

But with some proper wording, you can get them to eat very good food choices without making them feel like they're eating "health food," or anything that doesn't taste good.

SUPPLEMENTS

Justin,

How many servings are in a bottle of Metabotrop? I know it contains 120 capsules, but do I take 1 capsule a day?

Thanks.

---

2 capsules is a serving.

So if you're using it for pre-workout intensity/energy/stimulation, it is good for 60-120 workouts.

If you're using it for fat burning, you'll start out at 1 capsule a.m. and mid-afternoon or pre-workout and build up to 2 capsules 2x a day. Those trying to get into contest shape may want to build up to 2 capsules 3x a day over a long ramp-up period.

In this case, it is about a month to 2-month supply, depending on how quickly you ramp up the dosage.

Justin,

What are your thoughts on the best time to use Gemma Protein Isolate?

The best times are probably first thing in the morning and before and after workouts.

The best time is really anytime your blood amino pools will be lower and/or times when you need to spike blood amino pools rapidly.

Justin,

What is your opinion regarding cycling creatine? I was taking ethyl-ester creatine, and was on it for about 4-5 months. Do you feel it is necessary to take time off of creatine? Plus, I have been taking 4-6 g of taurine and arginine each day, split before and after my workout, with a multivitamin being taken before.

Thanks.

I see no reason for cycling the creatine. Once the creatine phosphate stores are saturated, you've pretty much reached your potential for intracellular fluid levels and creatine phosphate available for energy purposes. By stopping creatine, you will lose those levels but I don't know that you'll see any super compensation of creatine stores when you go back on.

I cycle mine out of laziness. From time to time I get bored with adding a bunch of things to my post-workout shake, or sometimes my creatine falls behind the washer. But, I don't necessarily decide the cycle length for creatine.

Justin,

Hey, I just watched your DVD and I'm very impressed with both the training and nutrition content. I'm sorry to give you another WMS question, but you seem to be the only real expert on it. Christian Thibaudeau wrote this on T-nation.com:

"I'm not saying that vitargo isn't good. In fact, when taken by itself, vitargo (waxy maize) is probably the best carb to quickly refill muscle glycogen. BUT, (and that is a big but) the reason for that superiority is lost as soon as it's taken with something else.

You see, vitargo/waxy maize is good because of its molecular weight, which makes it absorbable 80% faster than regular carb powder. However, when you mix it with other ingredients like amino acids, protein, creatine, etc., the combined molecular weight of the product becomes "normal" and the mixture is thus not absorbed any faster than other carbs/amino acids/protein formulas.
So in that regard it isn't worse and it isn't better... it's just more expensive."

I was wondering if it is true that mixing the WMS with other nutrients will lower the molecular weight. If so, is this why you usually separate your WMS and protein into 2 different shakes? Additionally, I'm a broke college student, so affording a lot of WMS could be a problem. Would mixing maltodextrin with WMS be a bad idea because of the previously quoted statement? If so, would I be able to get away with drinking some WMS and Anatrop in one shake and then malto with protein in another?

Thanks in advance for any advice.

I've kind of been saying the same thing since day one with WMS....I think I may have created a bit too much hype with that though.

I don't know of any studies showing the molecular weight of a combined meal of protein and WMS...so to say that it becomes 'normal' is really just an assumption.

Most amino-based nutrients have a much lower molecular weight and higher osmolality than WMS. But I don't know if that molecular weight is enough to offset the extremely high molecular weight of the WMS...and make the meal isotonic. I still believe you will get increased absorption rate even when WMS is mixed with other nutrients, and especially when WMS is mixed with liquid protein and highly bio-available amino acids.

I've done experiments on myself and it seems that there isn't a huge change in the gastric clearance rate. And as long as the protein is kept to a lower portion (less than 1/3 the gram amount of the WMS), I haven't noticed any real change at all. This is one of the main reasons I developed Anatrop. It has the specific nutrients critical to the stimulus of anabolism but is low enough in gram total that it is unlikely to cause a huge disruption in the absorption rate of WMS. I actually designed it to go WITH WMS.

A fellow by the name of Layne Norton posted something on WMS that talked about how WMS structure is that of many "branches." These branches allow for a larger surface area of sugar molecules that can be 'cleaved' from the WMS at any given time. This is another reason WMS can cause such a rapid uptake, despite it not being a sugar.
Compare this to maltodextrin, and its singular plane of glucose molecules that only allow one to be 'cleaved' at a time.

That was a very faint paraphrase of Layne's, so I may have not given it justice, but it seems that is another benefit of the rapid uptake of WMS besides its low osmolality.

Justin,

What are your thoughts on MicroLactin? A trainer at my Gym told me to take it.

Thanks for any advice.

Unless I see the ingredients and how it
"maximizes the body's natural anti-inflammatory system," I don't know that I think much of it.

I've looked at a few sites and I can't find the ingredients or nutrient breakdown of the product.

I would assume from the words "grass fed," that the protein in the product has a higher amount of Omega 3 and possibly Omega 6 fatty acids than milk protein from a feed lot heifer...

If that is the case, then I'd just buy some fish oil and borage oil.

Justin,

I just saw your product ANATROP and was wondering whether you recommend taking it by itself in water post-workout or would it be okay to mix it with protein and carbs in a post-workout drink?
Also, would you recommend it for post-weight training sessions only or would you also recommend it after high intensity cardio sessions too?

In the offseason, I use it pre, during, and post-workout.
So, I have it with a shake right before the gym, I sip on it during training, and I have another immediately post-workout.

It mixes great with waxy maize and is the exact nutrient blend I recommend with waxy maize.
When dieting, I have it with my post-workout and post-cardio meals.
If I have whole food, I mix it in Crystal Light (even though it is flavored, it has a bit of a bitter taste...pure BCAA's and L-taurine have that taste).

Remember to count the calories in it though.

If you mix it with chocolate whey protein, strawberry, or fruit punch waxy maize and a dab of fruit punch sugar free Kool-Aid, it tastes like a Tootsie Pop......at least to me. But, that could be because I've been dieting and anything tastes good.

Justin,

What are your thoughts on Vitargo? How does it compare to WMS for post-workout nutrition?

Vitargo is a decent product.

I think their formula changed a year or two ago to include a barley product instead of a waxy maize product.
You could tell the difference in texture.

It is still a HMW carbohydrate I'd imagine, but I prefer the use of waxy maize.

Justin,

Your amino blend Anatrop looks great! I am going to pick some up, but I'm not sure how many servings are in each container and what the exact measurements of the formula are. How would you use it when dieting down (i.e. servings and timing of the servings)?

Thanks.

It is a mix of BCAA's, extra L-leucine, creatine and L-taurine.

A full serving has 10g of BCAA's, with 5g extra L-leucine (for 10g total), 2g L-taurine, and 5g creatine.
A single scoop has 5g BCAA's, with 5g total L-leucine, 1g L-taurine, and about 3g creatine.
There are 40 single scoop servings per container.

Remember that there are about 8-9g of protein per scoop and you need to count that towards your meal totals.
BCAA's are still amino acids, which are protein.

Justin,

I did not see creatine available on your supplement website. What kind of creatine do you recommend and where would you recommend buying it?

I actually do have creatine on my website
www.TroponinNutrition.com

I don't carry creatine as a solo product, but it is an ingredient in my product Anatrop.

Anatrop is the exact amino acid and nutrient mix you often see me recommend around my workouts.

It contains 5g of BCAA's, 5g of additional L-leucine (for 10g total), 5g of creatine, and 2g of L-taurine per serving.

Combining the Anatrop with a high molecular weight carbohydrate like Waxy Maize should help you in shuttling a higher ratio of the creatine you ingest to your muscles.

POWERLIFTING

Justin,

When you did your powerlifting meet, what was your food and supplement intake like the day of your meet? Will you make any changes next time around?

Thank you.

I brought 4 meals of steak and rice, which I didn't have time to eat. I sipped on a combo shake of waxy maize, whey isolate, BCAA's, and creatine throughout the meet. Steady intake all day, sipping right up until a minute or two before my lifts.

I will do the same in the future, but I will add some other strength/endurance assisting nutrients, along with some electrolytes.
I'm actually looking into developing a product with these ingredients.

Also for my next meet, I plan on:
A large breakfast with plenty of complex carbs, healthy fats, and protein.

A large meal in between bench and deads.

Smaller compact meals to munch on during warm-ups.

I'll sip the mixture I mentioned steadily throughout the meet to keep blood aminos and blood sugar levels elevated steadily.

Justin,

Do you think it would be beneficial for a powerlifter to clean up his diet with about the same amount of calories for eight to ten weeks before a meet?

Thanks.

Complex carbohydrates, essential fatty acids, and complete proteins will fuel the body and fuel training more effectively than saturated fat and sugar.

So, I do believe in focusing on the correct nutrients.

I'm not a "low" calorie guy. I believe in BIG eating, but eating big on the right foods is better than eating saturated fat and sugar.

The goal should be to turn your body into a nutrient processing machine. But, to do this you have to give the body nutrients, not junk.

Justin,

Right now I compete in PL in the 220 class. Currently I weigh 215lbs. I recently tested my body fat with cheap calipers and also with a weight scale that uses bioelectrical impedance analysis. The results were 14% and 21% respectively. Needless to say, I need to get leaner.

My goal is to be 190lbs at 5% body fat by November 2007 for a powerlifting meet, and then dehydrate the rest to make 181lbs at weigh ins.

In the past I have gone from 192lbs at 17% body fat to 172lbs at 5% body fat over 6 months by bodybuilding training 5 days a week, with cardio 3 days a week, a solid thermogenic, a high protein diet consisting of whole foods and no processed carbs. Now that I compete in powerlifting, I am kind of lost on how to diet without losing strength. Currently I don't do any cardio and don't plan on using a thermogenic.

Can you make some recommendations on how I can achieve my goal?

Thanks in advance.

Joe

If you're interested in a more complete answer, you or anyone else who is interested can check out www.TroponinNutrition.com to see what I do, as well as see my nutritionists, and decide if they're right for you.

You were on the right path with the diet.
Keep the foods simple. Basic foods, good protein sources, complex carbs, and healthy fats are what you should focus on.

Rotate your calorie and carb amounts so that your highest carb intake is on heavy training days and your lowest carb intake is on off days.

Don't worry about cardio causing you to lose strength. You won't lose strength from just walking around for awhile on a treadmill. If anything, the increased capillary density and ability to transfer and assimilate oxygen and energy by the muscles will help your strength.

Don't try to drop the weight too quickly, but make certain that you're making progress each week.

Justin,

After a couple days of no carbs and sweating to drop weight to make a weigh-in for a powerlifting meet, what are the most important things to have directly after the weigh-ins to be on track for the rest of the day to get the weight back?

I'll probably be dropping from 205lbs to 198lbs.

Water and sodium are the most important things.

You need to restore glycogen levels and bring as much hydration to the body as possible.

Water and sodium will have the biggest effect on total weight and water volume in the body, both intracellular and extracellular.

You also need carbs. Carbs are what restore muscle glycogen and are very important for weight training, as they are the 'gasoline' for the body's engine.

In order for glycogen storage to occur, 3 things are required. These are glucose (obviously), water, and sodium.

So, to bring your weight up quickly and to bring as much water in the body as possible, load up on water, salt, and carbs.

I know many people use Gatorade, but if you use Gatorade be careful of stomach problems. The osmolality of Gatorade is quite high and the sugar content is a bit too high as well.

Drinking only Gatorade will cause you to feel bloated, as water pools in the stomach, which is not what you want when trying to eat a lot.

I actually like to use Gatorade at ½ strength. Just mix it 50/50 with water. This provides a lower osmolality and less rapid influx of blood sugar.

I also recommend a product called waxy maize, which is a high molecular weight carbohydrate. It does NOT sit in the stomach and has a very low osmolality that allows it to pull water through the stomach and be taken up into the muscle.

My own personal approach would be to eat a high salt diet (probably heavily salting my protein intake 'meat'), a VERY high water intake, and frequent high carb meals.

The waxy maize would be used in between meals throughout the day with a very high water intake along with the WM.

The ½ strength Gatorade would be taken (½ Gatorade, ½ water) with the whole food meals.

In case anyone is interested in how glycogen is stored, here's the basic run-down.

It is actually an 11-step process.
The first step is glucose-1-phosphate and uridine triphosphate combine with water to create uridine diphosphate and 2pi.

The next main step is the uridine diphosphate is transferred to a hydroxyl group of an existing chain, which forms the alpha 1,4 glycosidic link.

This is all activated by phosphoprotein phosphatase, which is activated by insulin.

So, the carbs raise insulin levels. The insulin raises phosphoprotein phosphatase. Phosphoprotein phosphatase activates glycogen synthesis.

I'll leave the insulin alone, but you can see why that is an important hormone in this process.

TRAINING

Justin,

Every once in awhile, I start to really burn out after about four weeks of training. Then for a week or two, my energy level is at zero. I know that my CNS is wrecked when this happens. My question is, when I get to this point would it be pointless to even go to the gym? Should I go and keep the weight super light, even below normal warm-up weight? Also, is there anything I can do to speed up the neural recovery besides eating and sleep? I am 18 years old.

Thanks,

Matt

I don't like to get too much into the over-training stuff. I feel people begin to listen too closely to their bodies and start to think they're over-trained as soon as they're not drooling with excitement for the next workout.

Your body will let you know when it is time to back off.
Your heart rate will become elevated in the mornings.
Your motivation will suffer.
You may get headaches.
You may get one of any number of other symptoms.

Don't fear hard work or worry that you're working too hard. I'm not saying that you've said this....but I'm tired of hearing people talk about working too hard.

As if they have to be extra careful not to work TOO hard or they'll shrivel up.
As if hard work is bad.
If I'm going to lean to one side, I'd rather work too hard than not hard enough.

I tend to focus on bodybuilding, as that is my main basis of training knowledge.
But, I hear hundreds of little guys talking about taking "a scoop of whey, glutamine, and some BCAA's" before cardio so they don't "lose muscle."

Or worrying about doing cardio too intensely so they don't "lose muscle."

Or worrying about training too hard so they don't get "over-trained."

While they're taking in 70g of protein before a short little walk on the treadmill in the morning, Ronnie Coleman is doing 2 HOURS a day on the stepmill at 300lbs.

Ronnie Coleman: trains 6x a week...each body part 2x a week, HEAVY weights, 2 hours of cardio pre-contest.

Jay Cutler: does as much as 40 sets for back...2x a day! Trains 2x a day, 5x a week.

Johnny 185-lb at the gym: stops after 6 sets, and is scared of cardio.

Check out Brian Sider's training routine. Whenever someone posts it online, the first thing people jump in on is, "That's TOO MUCH WORK!"

Don't be afraid of work. But when your body tells you it's time to back off, back off a little. But, if you're fired up to train, go at it.

Justin,

**I was just curious what your opinion is on scheduled time off.
I usually just take every third or forth day off or just rest when
I want. But lately I hear people saying I should take a
scheduled week off every 8 to 10 weeks. I tried it and took 7
days off and felt fine within 3 to 4 days.**

I ALWAYS plan on taking weeks off during the year.

But...I never actually take them off.

I just can't do it. Proper rest and recuperation is something I've
been focusing on in recent years. For years I would never take
more than a day or two off from the gym in a row.

It is important for the body to have periods of decreased workload
to allow for rejuvenation of the Central Nervous System.

Part of the reason I don't take enough time off is that I love to
train. If I have free time, I enjoy using it to train.

In recent times, I've become extremely busy with work, and have
been forced to take periods of decreased training frequency in
order to catch up on projects. I've realized that this isn't
necessarily a bad thing for me. When I come back from a few
weeks of moderate training intensity, I feel much better and get
more productive workouts.

Justin,

Since you're a pro bodybuilder and seem to know a lot in that area, I have a quick question for you. Do you have to be super strong to build muscle mass? In other words, can you use light weight to build muscle?

Thanks.

I'm not a pro bodybuilder...but thanks for the compliment!

You do not have to be super strong to build muscle mass.

Muscle mass is more than just contractile tissue.
Muscle is also composed of blood vessels, capillary beds, glycogen stores, sodium and other electrolyte stores, water, etc., etc.

The actual myosin and actin cross-sectional area is a relatively small portion of the total muscle 'size.'

Hypertrophy is caused by more than just elevated weight loads against its tension.

It is a long, complicated, and boring argument really.

Gaining strength will assist you in adding size. And no massive bodybuilder is weak by the average person's standards.

But ultimately, strength for sports like powerlifting doesn't require maximum levels of hypertrophy.

BUT...show me a small person who can:
bench 600lbs raw
squat 800lbs raw
deadlift 700lbs raw

Justin,

I wrote to you awhile ago expressing my new-found admiration of DC training. I have been doing more reading and stumbled upon an article where the author would "pop the scapula," which would enable his client to get a 1-3 inch larger lat spread. This sounded painful but the author wouldn't reveal any more secrets.

Do you know what I'm talking about? Have you done this? What exactly do they mean?

I know about the VERY secretive "scapula pop."

Unfortunately, its secrets have been kept even from me.

Dante actually says it's very hard to explain, and has tried to explain it a bit...

I'm going to San Diego in a few weeks to meet with everyone from the Trueprotein.com crew...I'll be sure to ask for more info on this.

Remind me in a few weeks, and I'll see if I have more info.

One thing that has really worked for me with lat spread is DEEP stretching of the lat following lat work.
I've rarely crossed a door in the last year without grabbing somewhere near the top and stretching my lat, trying to force my scapula out.

I honestly believe it has helped a ton.
You can look into traction and band work for this as well.

Justin,

I train for Powerlifting and Strongman. My days usually look like this:
day 1 Maximum Effort upper body
day 2 Dynamic Effort lower body
day 3 off
day 4 Dynamic Effort upper body
day 5 Maximum Effort lower body
day 6 off.
I train 2 days on, 1 day off. Currently, my low carb days are on my off days. My high carb days are on day 1 and day 4. The medium day is on day 2 and day 5.
Is this how you would set it up? My thought is that I need the extra recovery on the first training day so as to allow me to train harder on the second training day.

Thanks.

That is pretty much exactly how I would set it up.
You get the needed glycogen after a low day on that first high day. That glycogen will carry you through the second training day when calories are a bit lower. And the increased essential fatty acids and protein on low day will fuel growth on your rest days.

You should be able to stay lean, or even lose fat, as you gain strength.

Justin,

**During your pre-contest preparations, do you drop DC
training and go to a more traditional bodybuilding routine?**

When preparing for the 2007 USA's, I moved to a more traditional
routine initially. I travel a lot and my training partner was in
preparations to move to Texas, so he was away a lot.
We were having a hard time being on schedule with our training,
and weren't getting together to train very often.
When I don't have a partner, it is harder for me to follow the DC
program.

Once I found a consistent training partner, I returned to a DC type
training program.

DC training can be done without a spotter, but I prefer to use free
weights over machines and smith machines. DC training on free
weights without a spotter requires more care.

Justin,

You recommended DC training to me when I wanted a break from my normal routine. I love it! Thanks for the suggestion! Also, my wife is a former powerlifter, recording a 380lb bench press at 190lbs. She has converted to bodybuilding and won her first show, winning her class and the overall! She is getting a little more serious and she was wondering if you train people on-line, and if so, how would we contact you?

Thanks.

I do train people online. You can check us out at www.TroponinNutrition.com

Tell your wife congratulations, and I would love to work with her!

DC training is a very innovative training program that is fun to do. I enjoy training heavy and pushing myself.

You get both of those in spades with DC training.

Justin,

1) After coming off a de-load week 1 month ago, I decided to try 4 weeks of DC training and convinced my training partners to try it as well.

It is much more difficult than I had expected!
I had to increase my caloric intake by about 500 calories per day to keep up. I have a new-found respect for body builders.

2) What's your opinion on NO2 supplements?
One of my training partners swears by them pre-workout, but the only results I have personally experienced were having an increased micturation reflex 1-1.5 hours after taking them.
So, I was basically running to the restroom when I got to the gym.

---

1) It is definitely more work than people would think, especially when you're stronger and moving heavier weight than a beginning trainer.
It is only 1 all-out rest pause set, but the warm-ups it takes to get to a 600lb squat or deadlift is more involved than the warm-ups it would take to get to a 250lb squat.

If you put your all into it, it is a very good, and very tough program.

2) I think they're a bit over-hyped, and do little in the way of increasing muscle mass or strength.
Much of what people feel is psychological with the NO2 supplements. Vasodilation combined with stimulants is going to make you feel really good during your workout. You're going to be very energetic and you will feel more vascular.
It can be argued that the increase in vasodilation creates an environment for better shuttling of growth-promoting nutrients to the working muscle. I am a proponent of this effect when training and much of my workout nutrition protocol is planned around this

phenomenon.

However, I don't believe there is necessarily a need for increased vasodilation to receive this benefit. The body's natural adaptation to training is to create dilation of blood vessels leading to the working muscle. So, your body's natural function does what these products intend to do.

That isn't to say there is no benefit to their use, however. If they are proven to increase the availability of blood into the working muscle, it should create the environment for increased nutrient uptake by that muscle.

But, it isn't the first thing I would spend money on in a supplement.

Justin,

When your cardio is cranked up during pre-contest dieting, do you back off on your leg training volume? Do you keep the weights high or do you lighten it up and keep higher volume?

I do my normal weight training.

I don't change anything.

I actually find that my leg size seems to increase slightly, along with my training intensity as the cardio improves my recovery in the beginning.

I try like hell to use the same weights, or heavier, during my diet as I do in the offseason.

Justin,

I just finished your article about nutrition on t-nation.com and your training philosophy really caught my eye.

I have been lifting consistently for about 2.5 years. Up until three months ago, I utilized a more bodybuilding-style approach to training. But recently I have been using the Westside template to build strength. It has worked great in the short period of time I have used it, but I feel like my hypertrophy goals are falling behind now.

I do realize that training for strength and power is a different goal than training purely for hypertrophy, but you seem to manage both quite well.

My question is this: could you elaborate on your training methods and the various ways you combine powerlifting training with bodybuilding-style training?

Thanks,

Mike

You're going to be much less intrigued than you anticipated, I'm afraid.

Most of the time I just do a basic DC type approach.
DC focuses on strength gains, with rest pause techniques.

For the most part, I train for hypertrophy, but love lifting heavy. So, I tend to use as heavy of a weight as I can in a rep range designed for hypertrophy. For me, that means roughly 6 to 20 repetitions per set.

The biggest thing is that I try to achieve a goal every workout.

If I'm training DC, that goal is beating the log book on at least one movement.

If I'm not training DC, then it is doing something I think is fun every workout.

One recent workout was an attempt at 315lbs for 30 reps on bench. I also tried 225lbs for 60 reps in that workout.

Another recent workout was doing very deep Olympic-style squats with 585.

Some past workouts are trying 500lbs for 20 on squats, trying 50 reps on hack squats, and doing sets of 100 reps on leg presses.

I have a goal every workout, and try to reach it.

Do that each workout and be consistent with your eating for a dozen years or so, and you'll be both strong and large.

Justin,

I am new to the DC style of training and I was under the impression that you have some experience with it.

I am training a client who is not new to lifting weights but has never trained very intensely. Do you think it would be better to train him one body part 5 days a week, as he would prefer, or do you think that I could get more results for him with DC training?

Also, on the DC training, do you follow the slow eccentrics (8s/10s) for all of the warm-ups getting up to the main set?

Thanks for all the help and keep up the good work.

Hans

Hans,
I don't know where the slow eccentric information comes from.
As far as I know, that is 'internet hype' and has been blown out of proportion.

I don't believe Dante recommends that long of a negative--only that you control the weight.

In the end, whatever routine allows your client to train with the most enjoyment and intensity is what is going to produce the best results.
There is no question that I am a fan of DC style training.
It is everything that forces muscle growth. DC focuses on intense training sessions, deep stretching, and big eating.

Be very careful where you get your info on DC training.
If you've ever played the game "telephone" in elementary school, you would understand.

Much of what is spread as DC training around the net isn't 2nd or 3rd hand information, it's 5th, 10th, 50th hand information, and far off what is the real info.

For real DC information, you can check out www.intensemuscle.com where the DC creator, Dante, has a section devoted to DC training.

You can also check out my training DVD "Project Superheavyweight" at www.TroponinNutrition.com as it follows me through a full training cycle of DC training, along with a nutritional DVD free of charge.

Justin,

I bought your DVD and had a couple questions.

1) The three day split you perform on the DVD—were those the only days you worked out in a 7 day period? (e.g. Mon-Wed-Fri)

2) As far as a row movement, is the only time you do a rowing movement when you do a widowmaker set after a back width exercise?

---

1) We train 4x a week. So the first workout of the week gets repeated. This allows us to hit a few body parts 2x a week, and the others 1x a week. Each week different muscle groups get hit twice, while the others get a rest of only 1 session that week.

2) We include bent rows and T-bar rows frequently in our back thickness movements, but deadlifts and rack deads are our favorite thickness movements.

Those workouts were just 3 days of us in the gym. Our movements vary often, but we pretty much stick to the basics, just like you saw on the DVD.

Justin,

After watching your video, I had a question about your application of DC training.

Until now, I have always warmed up by going up to heavy single before going for reps. The result is that I can exert much greater power after going heavier. An example would be that I would be able to squat 365 for 20 on the way down, versus maybe only 5 reps on the way up. If trying DC training, would you recommend that I go heavy first to warm up or just start trying to improve without going heavy?

Thanks,

Duane

DC training is a bit different than powerlifting training.
To take squats as an example, the point of the movement is muscle growth, not necessarily the amount of weight lifted.
The way I build up is this:
I start with 135lbs and add a plate each set, taking none of the sets to failure, or even that close to it, although I won't typically go less than 5 reps per set.

When I reach the peak weight that I am planning on lifting for 4-8 reps, I do my first set. This is my main set.
Since rest-pausing on squats is potentially dangerous, I then do a back-off set after a minute or two of rest. In this set, I shoot for 10-12 reps with the most weight I can handle in that range. I then finish with a 'widowmaker' set of 20 reps after another few minutes of rest.
So, in essence, I am doing the same thing you are. My widowmaker set is usually something in the 400's, which is a weight I also passed on the way up, although I probably only did that weight for about 5 reps when warming up to my heaviest weights.

Justin,

Just wondering what exercises really hammer the vastus medialis? I don't get much in the way of development with this muscle.

Thanks.

It's going to be tough to isolate a singular muscle in the quadriceps. They all work synergistically to extend the knee and to flex the hip flexors, moving the femur at the hip.

But, most EMG analyses shows that leg extensions with toes pointed out, so that the vastus medialis is pointed upwards away from the floor, create an environment where more stimulus is placed on that muscle.

Wider stance squatting and leg press movements have also been shown to create an increased activity on that muscle.

It is my own personal belief and experience that those with a vastus medialis that inserts very close to the knee, as opposed to higher up on the leg, get a higher rate of muscle activity there. So it is likely that your particular muscular insertions may be involved in your development issues.

I also feel an increase in lactic acid buildup when I do movements where my knees travel out past my toes, and also when I go very deep. But, this may be due primarily to the increase in stretch on the vastus medialis creating tightness in that area which will not allow as much blood flow out of that muscle, especially at the very bottom of the movement. This would create an environment almost like tourniquet training.

Justin,

**I have always had trouble getting my lats bigger. What would you suggest I do? I'm thinking about trying to do some really high volume stuff like lat pulldowns before I do deadlifts.
Do you have any suggestions?**

Thanks.

I was in the same boat for years...my lats were horrible.

I spoke with Dante Trudel of DC training fame, and we talked about a few unique exercises.

The main exercise is rope seated rows. They're a bit difficult to explain, so I hope this makes sense.

Use the rope handle, and use it on the seated row.

Sit way back on the bench, with your feet on the floor. Lean all the way over as far over as you can.

You don't even have to arch your back—a little upper back rounding is fine.

Pull the rope down to your waist, keeping your upper body as far forward as you can.
You will be forced to use much less weight than you would use in the standard seated row.

I prefer to use a rep range of 15-20 repetitions.

Really focus on letting the scapula spread at the top, and a strong contraction at the bottom.
This is the only exercise where I can totally isolate my lats. I get a very good pump, which I feel has allowed me to create better innervation with the lat muscles. This has allowed me to increase

my latissimus dorsi activity on other movements as well.

After the set is done, and the blood starts rushing in, do deep painful stretching of your lats. To perform this stretch, grab something and pull your arm over head and stretch your lats by spreading your scapula. I try to hold this stretched position for 60 seconds or more.

When you're done, you should feel blood rush into the area.

Stretch your lats after each set, and stretch the fascial tissue surrounding the muscle. This should allow more blood to flow into the muscle.

This allows you to focus on the "BIG" movements for back the rest of the workout. The heavy compound movements add the most size. You can focus on just a few sets of this one particular exercise to hit your lats.

Justin,

Do you feel that the clean and press has helped your bench at all? I was thinking about adding the press to my DB cleans, and I noticed that you're one of a few lifters who do them on a consistent basis.

Thanks for your time and answer.

I'm not sure if it helps my bench or not.
Until I decided to compete in powerlifting, I hadn't done bench presses with any regularity in years.
I'm fairly sure it isn't a detriment to my bench press strength.

I think it probably aids in deadlift as well, as the clean portion mimics the biomechanics of a speed deadlift for many of the muscles involved.

Standing press is harder than seated press, and clean and press is harder than standing press.
I'm a person who believes that hard work pays off, and an exercise is hard for a reason. It is usually harder because it is working more muscle tissue.

I don't include them every workout, but I include them pretty frequently.

Justin,

I've seen you quoted as, "First of all, I find that moderate cardio actually increases my lifts."

What is "moderate cardio" for you?

Thanks.

I do about 20 minutes of fairly high intensity 4x a week in the offseason, immediately after my workout.

I don't do it for fat burning, as I have plenty of carbohydrates in me from my pre-workout shake, and also from my during-workout shake.

I do it for overall health benefits and the increased cardiovascular capacity, which can help drive through heavy training.

I notice the largest cardiovascular benefit for leg movements. With a lot of weigh on your back, your lungs can almost give out before your legs.

Doing the cardio helps me utilize the oxygen a bit better and make sure my legs are what fatigues first.

Justin,

How do you do a Romanian deadlift?

This is how "I" do them.
I keep my back arched, especially my lower back.
My legs are stiff, but not locked straight. There is a slight bend in the knees. I keep my head looking forward, and not down.

I bend over by sinking back on my hips, and keeping that arch in my back.
I find that I can only get the bar to about mid-shin level before my back starts to round.

Romanian deadlifts are a great hamstring, glute, and lower back exercise.

Justin,

How often do you train for pure strength and how long does that period last? How does your training differ in preparation for a powerlifting meet compared to your regular offseason bodybuilding training? Do you try and stay lean year-round?

Good luck in your future goals.

As of now, I haven't really trained for pure strength.
I've always enjoyed training heavy, but my training since 2001 has been 100% for bodybuilding.
I trained for football until I finished playing in college, so that training was geared towards strength and explosion.

My training didn't really differ when training for my first powerlifting meet.

I changed things some, as I was training DC at the time.
I really just did my normal routine, but added an extra session each week to do wide stance squats.
My other leg day was a normal leg training session for me.

I also tried my bench shirt on arm day, but I only got to try it 3 times before the meet.

In the future, I will definitely put more concentrated efforts into a powerlifting meet.

I will always train with bodybuilding in mind, but I will devote more time to learning equipment and maximizing leverage with my form.

I do try to stay lean year round. I don't see the benefit in gaining fat. Most studies show the human body to be most anabolic at a lower fat range.
It also makes it easier to get in shape for a contest when I'm only

trying to lose 10lbs of fat and 5-10lbs of water.
I am very meticulous with my diet year round, so the opportunity to gain fat never really comes up.